ABC of
Geriatric Medicine

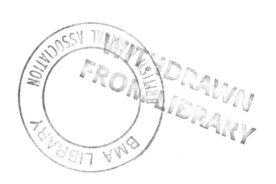

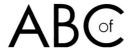

ABC of

Geriatric Medicine

EDITED BY

Nicola Cooper

Consultant in Acute Medicine and Geriatrics
Leeds General Infirmary
Great George Street
Leeds, LS1 3EX

Kirsty Forrest

Consultant in Anaesthesia and Education
Leeds General Infirmary
Great George Street
Leeds, LS1 3EX

Graham Mulley

Professor of Elderly Medicine and President of the British Geriatrics Society
Consultant in Elderly Medicine, Leeds Primary Care Trust and
Department of Elderly Medicine
St James's University Hospital
Leeds, LS9 7TF

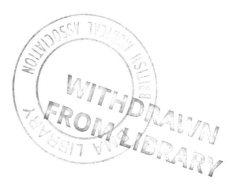

WILEY-BLACKWELL

A John Wiley & Sons, Ltd., Publication

BMJ|Books

This edition first published 2009, © 2009 by Blackwell Publishing Ltd

BMJ Books is an imprint of BMJ Publishing Group Limited, used under licence by Blackwell Publishing which was acquired by John Wiley & Sons in February 2007. Blackwell's publishing programme has been merged with Wiley's global Scientific, Technical and Medical business to form Wiley-Blackwell.

Registered office: John Wiley & Sons Ltd, The Atrium, Southern Gate, Chichester, West Sussex, PO19 8SQ, UK

Editorial offices: 9600 Garsington Road, Oxford, OX4 2DQ, UK
The Atrium, Southern Gate, Chichester, West Sussex, PO19 8SQ, UK
111 River Street, Hoboken, NJ 07030-5774, USA

For details of our global editorial offices, for customer services and for information about how to apply for permission to reuse the copyright material in this book please see our website at www.wiley.com/wiley-blackwell

The right of the author to be identified as the author of this work has been asserted in accordance with the Copyright, Designs and Patents Act 1988.

Wiley also publishes its books in a variety of electronic formats. Some content that appears in print may not be available in electronic books.

Designations used by companies to distinguish their products are often claimed as trademarks. All brand names and product names used in this book are trade names, service marks, trademarks or registered trademarks of their respective owners. The publisher is not associated with any product or vendor mentioned in this book. This publication is designed to provide accurate and authoritative information in regard to the subject matter covered. It is sold on the understanding that the publisher is not engaged in rendering professional services. If professional advice or other expert assistance is required, the services of a competent professional should be sought.

The contents of this work are intended to further general scientific research, understanding, and discussion only and are not intended and should not be relied upon as recommending or promoting a specific method, diagnosis, or treatment by physicians for any particular patient. The publisher and the author make no representations or warranties with respect to the accuracy or completeness of the contents of this work and specifically disclaim all warranties, including without limitation any implied warranties of fitness for a particular purpose. In view of ongoing research, equipment modifications, changes in governmental regulations, and the constant flow of information relating to the use of medicines, equipment, and devices, the reader is urged to review and evaluate the information provided in the package insert or instructions for each medicine, equipment, or device for, among other things, any changes in the instructions or indication of usage and for added warnings and precautions. Readers should consult with a specialist where appropriate. The fact that an organization or Website is referred to in this work as a citation and/or a potential source of further information does not mean that the author or the publisher endorses the information the organization or Website may provide or recommendations it may make. Further, readers should be aware that Internet Websites listed in this work may have changed or disappeared between when this work was written and when it is read. No warranty may be created or extended by any promotional statements for this work. Neither the publisher nor the author shall be liable for any damages arising herefrom.

Library of Congress Cataloging-in-Publication Data

ABC of geriatric medicine / edited by Nicola Cooper, Kirsty Forrest, Graham Mulley.
     p. ; cm.
   Includes bibliographical references and index.
   ISBN 978-1-4051-6942-4 (alk. paper)
   1. Geriatrics--Great Britain. I. Cooper, Nicola. II. Forrest, Kirsty. III. Mulley, Graham P.
   [DNLM: 1. Geriatrics--Great Britain. 2. Health Services for the Aged--Great Britain. WT 100 A112 2008]
   RC952.A25 2008
   618.97--dc22

                                                                              2008001980

ISBN: 978-1-4051-6942-4

A catalogue record for this book is available from the British Library.

Set in 9.25/12 pt Minion by Newgen Imaging Systems Pvt. Ltd, Chennai, India
Printed in Singapore by Ho Printing Singapore Pte Ltd

3   2013

Contents

Contributors

Eileen Burns
Consultant in Geriatric Medicine
Leeds General Infirmary, Leeds, UK

Jon Cooper
Consultant in Geriatrics and Stroke Medicine
Leeds General Infirmary, Leeds, UK

Nicola Cooper
Consultant in Acute Medicine and Geriatrics
Leeds General Infirmary, Leeds, UK

Stephen Curran
Professor of Old Age Psychopharmacology and
Consultant in Old Age Psychiatry
University of Huddersfield, UK

Mamoun Elmamoun
Senior House Officer in General Medicine
Leeds General Infirmary, Leeds, UK

Kirsty Forrest
Consultant in Anaesthesia and Education
Leeds General Infirmary, Leeds, UK

John Holmes
Senior Lecturer in Liaison Psychiatry of Old Age
Academic Unit of Psychiatry and Behavioural Sciences
Leeds University, UK

Julia Howarth
Advanced Clinical Pharmacist (Acute Hospital Care for Older People)
St James's University Hospital, Leeds, UK

Raja Hussain
Consultant in General Medicine and Geriatrics
Pinderfields General Hospital, Wakefield, UK

Suzanne Kite
Consultant in Palliative Care
Leeds General Infirmary, Leeds, UK

Graham Mulley
Professor of Elderly Medicine
Department of Elderly Medicine
St James's University Hospital, Leeds, UK

Lucy Nicholson
Specialist Registrar in Palliative Care
Yorkshire, UK

John Pearn
Senior House Officer in General Medicine
Leeds General Infirmary, Leeds, UK

Lauren Raltson
Specialist Registrar in General Medicine and Geriatrics
Yorkshire, UK

Anne Siddle
Specialist Nurse in Continence Care
St Mary's Hospital, Leeds, UK

Catherine Tandy
Consultant in Acute Hospital and Community Geriatrics
Leeds General Infirmary, Leeds, UK

Katrina Topp
Consultant in Orthogeriatrics
Leeds General Infirmary, Leeds, UK

Nicola Turner
Consultant in Acute Hospital and Community Geriatrics
St James's University Hospital, Leeds, UK

John Wattis
Professor of Old Age Psychiatry
University of Huddersfield, UK

John Young
Professor of Geriatric Medicine
Dept of Elderly Care, Bradford Teaching
Hospitals NHS Foundation Trust, UK

Rosemary Young
Medical Social Worker in Care of the Elderly
Leeds General Infirmary, Leeds, UK

Preface

Geriatric medicine is practised by many different clinicians in a wide variety of settings: hospital wards, outpatient clinics, day hospitals, general practitioner surgeries, care homes and the patient's own home.

Most doctors will spend a large part of their time dealing with older patients, which is why geriatric medicine is important. It is also a challenge: illness in older people often presents in atypical ways; and there is sometimes an inaccurate perception that little can be done to help them, or that their problems are 'social' rather than medical.

The *ABC of Geriatric Medicine* is written as an introduction to the specialty. The chapters are based on the UK's postgraduate curriculum for geriatric medicine and cover both general and specific aspects of medicine for older people, with further resources.

This book is for doctors in training – in hospital or general practice – and for medical students and specialist nurses. It can also be used as a resource for teaching. We hope you enjoy using it.

Interpretation of the text

The conditions discussed in this book refer specifically to older people and it should not be assumed that the same approach is relevant in younger patients, unless specifically stated.

The text and figures refer mainly to geriatric medicine in the UK; however, many of the principles apply to other developed countries.

Nicola Cooper
Kirsty Forrest
Graham Mulley

Acknowledgements

The editors would like to thank Mary Banks of Wiley-Blackwell for allowing this project to go ahead, and to the rest of the Wiley-Blackwell team for all their hard work. Thanks also go to the authors and to Dr Jon Martin, specialist registrar in radiology, Leeds, for his help in providing and interpreting radiological images for publication.

CHAPTER 1

Introducing Geriatric Medicine

Nicola Cooper & Graham Mulley

OVERVIEW

- Developed countries have an ageing population
- Sick old people often present differently to younger people and can be clinically complex
- Atypical presentations such as reduced mobility are not 'social' problems – they are medical problems in disguise
- Comprehensive geriatric assessment and rehabilitation are of central importance to geriatric medicine and have a strong evidence base
- Simple interventions can often make a big difference to the quality of life of an older person

---

Geriatric medicine is important because most doctors deal with older patients. In the UK, people over the age of 65 make up around 16% of the population, but this group accounts for 43% of the entire National Health Service (NHS) budget and 71% of social care packages. Two-thirds of general hospital beds are used by older people and they present to most medical specialties (Figure 1.1).

The proportion of older people is growing steadily (Figure 1.2), with even greater increases in the over 85 age group. According to official figures, the numbers of people aged 85 and over are projected to grow from 1.1 million in 2000 to 4 million in 2051.

Geriatric medicine is mainly concerned with people over the age of 75, although most 'geriatric' patients are much older. Many of these have several complex, interacting medical and psychosocial problems which affect their function and independence.

Age-related differences

There are important differences in the physiology and presentation of older people that every clinician needs to know about. These in turn affect assessment, investigations and management (Box 1.1).

Special features of illness in older people include the following.

Multiple pathology

Older people commonly present with more than one problem, usually with a number of causes. A young person with fever, anaemia,

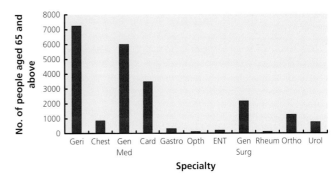

Figure 1.1 The numbers of people aged 65 and above admitted to a general hospital each year, by specialty. (Figures from the Leeds Teaching Hospitals NHS Trust.) Geri, geriatric medicine; Chest, chest medicine; Gen Med, general medicine; Card, cardiology; Gastro, gastroenterology; Opth, ophthalmology; ENT, ear, nose and throat; Gen Surg, general surgery; Rheum, rheumatology; Ortho, orthopaedics; Urol, urology.

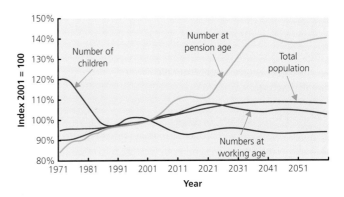

Figure 1.2 Changes in the proportion of people aged 65 and above among the overall population. Information from The UK National Census (2001).

a heart murmur and microscopic haematuria may have endocarditis, but in an older person this presentation is more likely to be due to a urinary tract infection, aspirin-induced gastritis and aortic sclerosis. Never stop at a single unifying diagnosis – always consider several.

Atypical presentation

Older people commonly present with 'general deterioration' or functional decline. Acute disease is often masked but precipitates

---

ABC of Geriatric Medicine. Edited by N. Cooper, K. Forrest and G. Mulley.
© 2009 Blackwell Publishing, ISBN: 978-1-4051-6942-4.

functional impairment in other areas. Therefore atypical presentations such as falls, confusion or reduced mobility are *not* social problems – they are medical problems in disguise (Box 1.2). Often the history has to be sought from relatives and carers, over the telephone if necessary.

Reduced homeostatic reserve

Ageing is associated with a decline in organ function with a reduced ability to compensate. The ability to increase heart rate and cardiac output in critical illness is reduced; renal failure due to medications or illness is more likely; salt and water homeostasis is impaired so electrolyte imbalances are common in sick older people; thermoregulation may also be impaired. In addition, quiescent diseases are often exacerbated by acute illness; for example heart failure may occur with pneumonia and old neurological signs may become more pronounced with sepsis.

Impaired immunity

Older people do not necessarily have a raised white cell count or a fever with infection. Hypothermia may occur instead. A rigid abdomen is uncommon in older people with peritonitis – they are more likely to get a generally tender but soft abdomen. Measuring the serum C-reactive protein can be useful when screening for infection in an older person who is non-specifically unwell.

Some clinical findings are not necessarily pathological

Neck stiffness, a positive urine dipstick in women, mild crackles at the bases of the lungs, a slightly reduced PaO_2 and reduced skin turgor may be normal findings in older people and do not always indicate disease.

The importance of functional assessment and rehabilitation

Older people may take longer to recover from illness (e.g. pneumonia) compared with younger people. However, their ability to perform activities of daily living and thus gain independence can improve dramatically if they are given time and rehabilitation.

Ethics

Geriatric medicine involves balancing the right to high-quality care without age discrimination with the wisdom to avoid aggressive and ultimately futile interventions. End-of-life decisions, risks vs benefits, capacity and consent, and dealing with vulnerable adults are all part of geriatric medicine.

In acute illness, the above factors combined can make clinical assessment very difficult and early intervention more important. For example, in severe sepsis, older patients may have cool peripheries and appear 'shut down', with a normal white cell count and no fever. Drowsiness is common, and does not necessarily indicate a primary brain problem. The patient may not be able to give a history, and their usual level of function and previously expressed wishes may not be known. Thus, gathering as much information as possible, as soon as possible, is vital.

Comprehensive geriatric assessment

In the 1930s, the very first geriatricians realised that the thousands of patients living in hospitals and workhouses were not suffering from 'old age' but from diseases that could be treated: immobility, falls, incontinence and confusion – called the 'geriatric giants' because they are the common presentations of different illnesses in older people (Box 1.3).

Today, geriatric medicine is the second biggest hospital specialty in the UK and a popular career choice. It involves dealing with acute illness, chronic disease and rehabilitation, working in multidisciplinary teams in the community and in hospitals, medical education and research.

Comprehensive geriatric assessment is the assessment of a patient made by a team which includes a geriatrician, followed by interventions and goal setting agreed with the patient and carers. This can take place in the community, in assessment areas linked to the emergency department, or in hospital. It covers the following areas:

- medical diagnoses
- review of medicines and concordance with drug therapy
- social circumstances
- assessment of cognitive function and mood
- functional ability (i.e. ability to perform activities of daily living; Box 1.4)
- environment
- economic circumstances.

Randomised controlled trials show that comprehensive geriatric assessment leads to improved function and quality of life, and also reduces hospital stay, readmission rates and institutionalisation. There is no evidence for the effectiveness of a comprehensive assessment that does not include a doctor trained in geriatric medicine.

Rehabilitation is an important aspect of geriatric medicine (see Chapter 11). Many older patients now have rehabilitation in intermediate care facilities or in their own homes. However, some of these patients undergo rehabilitation without the benefit of a comprehensive geriatric assessment, so that the opportunity for diagnosis, treatment and optimum rehabilitation may be lost.

Communication in geriatric medicine

Communication is particularly important in geriatric medicine. A history from the patient's relatives or carers is often required and may differ significantly from that of the patient. The assessment of older people often requires a multidisciplinary team and the observations, skills and opinions of nurses, physiotherapists, occupational therapists and social workers may shed significant new light on the patient's problems. Doctors who work with older people need to be comfortable with this multidisciplinary approach, and the often jigsaw puzzle-like progress in assessment that can sometimes occur.

Communicating with older patients may be difficult because of impaired vision, deafness, dysphasia or dementia. Healthcare professionals can aid communication by checking that the patient can hear what is being said, writing down instructions, and involving carers in the consultation and decision-making.

Simple interventions can make a big difference

Another characteristic of geriatric medicine is that simple interventions can make a big difference to a patient's function and quality of life. Sometimes there is a perception that 'nothing can be done' for very old people. This is rarely the case. For example:

- ear syringing, cataract surgery and a new pair of glasses can dramatically improve a person's sense of social isolation and loneliness
- specially fitted shoes and a properly measured walking aid can improve balance, mobility and confidence
- reducing medications can stop a person from feeling dizzy when they walk and allow them to go out of the house again
- adaptations at home can allow people to function more easily and retain their independence.

When older people have the benefit of medical assessment and treatment for problems which are often perceived as being due to old age (e.g. incontinence, falls, memory problems), they and their carers can enjoy a better quality of life.

The future directions of geriatric medicine

The National Service Framework (NSF) for Older People in England was published in 2001 (Figure 1.3). NSFs are long-term

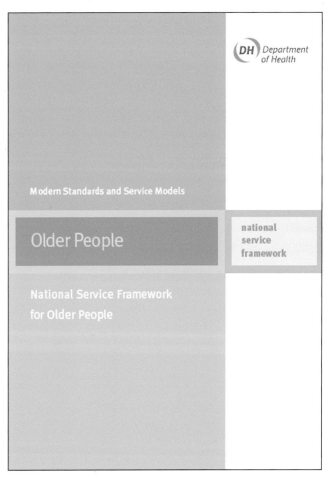

Figure 1.3 National Service Framework for Older People.

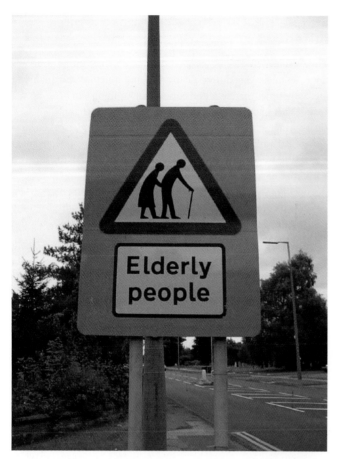

Figure 1.4 Elderly stereotypes. UK traffic sign showing a frail elderly couple.

strategies for improving specific areas of care, with funding, measurable goals and set time frames. The eight standards in the NSF for older people are:

- rooting out age discrimination
- person-centred care
- intermediate care
- general hospital care
- stroke
- falls
- mental health in older people
- promotion of health and active life in older age.

This has resulted in improved access to services, an increase in people having assessment and rehabilitation without the need to stay in hospital, and the development of specific age-related services (i.e. stroke and falls). More recently the Department of Health has launched 'dignity in care' which aims to improve key aspects of health and social services care for older people. It covers areas that older people and their carers consider to be important yet are often neglected.

- Being valued as a person (e.g. listened to, respected).
- Being given privacy during care.
- Having assistance with and enough time to eat meals.
- Being asked how one prefers to be addressed (e.g. whether by first name).
- Having services that are designed with older people in mind.

Considerable progress has been made in optimising the assessment and care of older people. However, the future still holds some challenges. These include how we can improve:

- the experience of older people in hospital and care homes
- access to comprehensive geriatric assessment in a variety of settings
- services for older people who present to the emergency department with falls, dementia and minor medical illnesses
- research that answers questions about important geriatric problems and processes of care.

Despite the persistence of some negative stereotypes (Figure 1.4), there is a great deal of variety and job satisfaction to be found in practising geriatric medicine, whether in hospital or in general practice. Older people *can* get better after assessment and treatment, and they are often very grateful for it.

Further resources

www.bgs.org.uk. The British Geriatrics Society website. For hospital doctors, general practitioners and specialist nurses working in geriatric medicine. Contains useful information about comprehensive geriatric assessment and other topics.

Nichol C, Wilson J, Webster S. (2008) *Lecture Notes on Elderly Care Medicine*, 7th edn. Blackwell Publishing, Oxford.

Rai GS, Mulley GP, eds. (2007) *Elderly Medicine: a Training Guide*, 2nd edn. Churchill Livingstone, London.

Department of Health. (2001) *National Service Framework for Older People*. DH, London.

www.dh.gov.uk. The UK Department of Health website. By using the search term 'older people' various relevant policy documents can be found.

CHAPTER 2

Prescribing in Older People

Jon Cooper & Julia Howarth

OVERVIEW

- Most older people are on regular medication
- Pharmacokinetics and pharmacodynamics are different in this age group
- Older people are much more likely to suffer from the side-effects of drugs
- Polypharmacy and problems with concordance are particular issues in geriatric medicine
- Drug trials tend not to include people over the age of 80

Two-thirds of people over the age of 60 are taking regular medication, and over half of those with repeat prescriptions are taking more than four drugs. People in care homes are even more likely to be taking several regular medications. Adverse drug reactions account for up to 17% of hospital admissions.

Pharmacokinetics and pharmacodynamics in old age

Pharmacokinetics refers to what the body does to a drug. Pharmacodynamics refers to what a drug does to the body.

Pharmacokinetic differences

Age-related changes lead to differences in absorption, distribution, metabolism and elimination of drugs. Whilst some of these differences are not clinically significant, some are.

- There is a reduced volume of distribution for many drugs because of reduced total body water and an increase in the percentage of body weight as fat. As a result, dose requirements are less than in younger people. For example, digoxin is a water-soluble drug, and lower loading doses may be required. Diazepam is a lipid-soluble drug and the relative increase in body fat may lead to accumulation, causing toxicity.
- Liver metabolism is reduced, leading to slower drug inactivation. Reduced liver blood flow is made worse by cardiac failure, potentially leading to increased drug concentrations, although this

is rarely of clinical significance. However, care should be taken when prescribing drugs that are metabolised in the liver and have a narrow therapeutic index: warfarin, theophyllines and phenytoin. Plasma levels of these drugs should be monitored.
- Perhaps the most clinically significant difference is that renal blood flow and mass reduce significantly with age, leading to a reduction in the clearance of many drugs, especially water-soluble ones. Because of less muscle mass, the creatinine can remain within the quoted normal range in older people, despite a significantly impaired glomerular filtration rate (GFR). Doses of some commonly prescribed drugs should be reduced to account for reduced renal function (as measured by GFR). Examples are ciprofloxacin, gentamicin, digoxin and lithium.

Pharmacodynamic differences

There is an increased sensitivity to drugs in general, and lower doses are often required compared to younger adults, primarily due to changes in drug receptors and impaired homeostatic mechanisms. For example, a patient started on treatment for hypertension may develop dizziness due to reduced baroreceptor sensitivity causing postural hypotension.

Adverse drug reactions

Adverse drug reactions (ADRs) are a common reason for hospital admission. Around 80% of ADRs are dose related, predictable and potentially preventable. Other ADRs may be allergic or idiosyncratic (unpredictable). However, ADRs often present in older patients non-specifically e.g. with confusion or falls.

Older people are more likely to have diseases that result in disease–drug interactions. Table 2.1 illustrates examples of diseases in old age and the disease–drug interactions that can occur with commonly prescribed medications. Every prescriber should consider these before prescribing for an older person.

There are a number of 'problematic' drugs in older people – prescribed medications that commonly cause side-effects. These are listed in Box 2.1.

Polypharmacy and drug–drug interactions

'Polypharmacy' is when a patient is taking a large number of different prescribed medications, some of which may be required, and

ABC of Geriatric Medicine. Edited by N. Cooper, K. Forrest and G. Mulley.
© 2009 Blackwell Publishing, ISBN: 978-1-4051-6942-4.

Disease in older age	Drugs	Potential effect
Dementia	Benzodiazepines Antimuscarinics, (some) anticonvulsants Levodopa	Worsening confusion
Parkinson's disease	Antimuscarinics Metoclopramide	Worsening symptoms Deteriorating movement disorder
Seizure disorder/epilepsy	Antibiotics Analgesics Antidepressants Antipsychotics Theophyllines Alcohol	Reduced seizure threshold/seizures
Glaucoma	Antimuscarinics	Worsening glaucoma
COPD/asthma	β-blockers Benzodiazepines	Bronchospasm Respiratory suppression
Heart failure	Diltiazem, verapamil NSAIDs	Worsening heart failure
Hypertension	NSAIDs, pseudoephedrine	Hypertension
Orthostatic hypotension	Antihypertensives (any) Diuretics Tricyclic antidepressants Levodopa	Postural hypotension Falls
Cardiac conduction disorders	β-blockers, digoxin, diltiazem, verapamil, amiodarone, Tricyclic antidepressants	Bradycardia, heart block, prolonged QTc
Peripheral arterial disease	β-blockers	Intermittent claudication
Peptic ulcer disease	NSAIDs, anticoagulants	Upper gastrointestinal haemorrhage
Hypokalaemia	Digoxin	Cardiac arrhythmia
Hyponatraemia	Diuretics Tricyclic antidepressants Carbamazepine	Worsening hyponatraemia May cause or exacerbate SIADH
Renal impairment	NSAIDS Antibiotics	Acute renal failure
Bladder outflow obstruction/ Benign prostate hyperplasia	Antimuscarinics α-blockers	Urinary retention
Urinary incontinence	α-blocker Antimuscarinics Benzodiazepines Diuretics Tricyclic antidepressants	Polyuria Worsening stress incontinence
Constipation	Antimuscarinics Calcium channel antagonists Tricyclic antidepressants Analgesics (e.g. opioids)	Worsening constipation
Osteoporosis	Steroids Enzyme inducing drugs	Accelerated osteoporosis

Table 2.1 Diseases in old age, and disease–drug interactions with commonly prescribed drug groups.

COPD, chronic obstructive pulmonary disease; NSAIDs, non-steroidal anti-inflammatory drugs; SIADH, syndrome of inappropriate antidiuretic hormone.

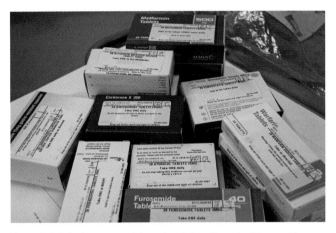

Figure 2.1 Polypharmacy and drug–drug interactions. An 86-year-old man with atrial fibrillation, heart failure, renal impairment and benign prostatic hypertrophy presents with dysuria. He has had several falls previously. He is prescribed ciprofloxacin based on previous urine sensitivities. This is an opportunity to review his medication. He takes twelve drugs regularly which are on repeat prescription, including:
- alfuzosin
- atenolol
- amiodarone
- perindopril
- furosemide
- warfarin.

He is on several medications that cause falls. Warfarin therapy may now be unsafe because of this. Ciprofloxacin interacts with warfarin and increases the risk of bleeding.

some not. There is no strict definition of polypharmacy, although the National Service Framework for Older People suggests a definition of being on four or more drugs. Some of the reasons for polypharmacy are listed in Box 2.2.

Taking a large number of different drugs is linked to adverse drug reactions, increased risk of hospital admission, non-compliance, and increased costs to the National Health Service. Figure 2.1 gives an example.

Drug–drug interactions become more likely with increasing number of medications. Herbal remedies and food can also interact with prescribed medication. A patient on warfarin for atrial fibrillation may develop bleeding after starting Gingko Biloba, a herbal medicine that inhibits platelet aggregation. A patient prescribed felodipine for hypertension may develop profound dizziness after drinking grapefruit juice, which increases drug levels.

Concordance

Concordance refers to the agreement between prescriber and patient about the goals of treatment and how such goals will be reached. Concordance is good when there is clear communication (Figure 2.2), understanding and agreement, and a drug regimen that is easy to follow, with packaging, labels and delivery systems that are easy to use. Compliance (or adherence) is the extent to which a person follows the prescriber's advice and drug regimen. Both concordance and compliance are particularly relevant to older people, although age itself is not a predictor of non-compliance. Box 2.3 lists some of the risk factors associated with poor compliance, and Box 2.4 shows the American Geriatric Society guidelines for providing information on medicines to patients.

The *ability* of an individual patient to administer a medicine should also be considered before prescribing. There are several

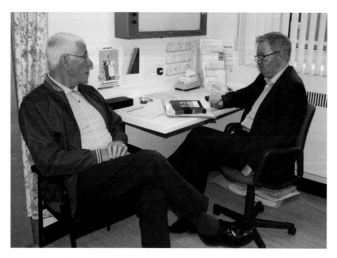

Figure 2.2 Communication and concordance.

Box 2.3 **Risk factors associated with non-compliance**

Risk factor	Association
Cognitive function	Strong
Health belief model	Strong
Polypharmacy	Strong
Not having home care services	Strong
Using more than one community pharmacy	Strong
Lifelong need for medication	Strong
Medication regime complexity	Strong
Side-effects experienced	Strong
Knowledge about medicines	Moderate
Poor recall of medicines being taken	Moderate
Female gender	Weak

Risk factors given in **bold type** are also correlated with the likelihood of hospital admission due to non-compliance. Col N, Fanale JE, Kronholm P. The role of medication non-compliance and adverse drug reactions in hospitalizations of the elderly. *Arch Intern Med* 1990; 170: 841–5.

Other factors influencing non-compliance include a poor relationship with the prescriber and insufficient time allowed for the consultation.

Reproduced with permission from Armour D, Cairns C, eds. (2002) *Medicines in the Elderly*. Pharmaceutical Press, London

---

strategies (e.g. Dossett box, inhaler aids) that can be employed to assist people with medicine-taking. Many of these can be advised by a pharmacist.

Evidence-based prescribing in older people

There is an increasing evidence base for drug management in older patients with diseases that are more prevalent with old age (e.g. atrial fibrillation, hypertension, heart failure, stroke and high cholesterol). However, applying evidence-based medicine to *all* older patients is not necessarily appropriate for a number of

---

Box 2.4 **Information to give patients to improve compliance**

About a specific medicine
Name of the drug
Purpose of the drug
Dose or 'strength'
When to be taken in relation to food or other medicines
Common side-effects
How long to take medicine for
Other warnings

General information about medicines
Do not take someone else's tablets
Keep taking medicine at the prescribed dose unless otherwise directed
Do not transfer medicines into an inappropriate container
Avoid taking your medicines in the dark

From: American Geriatric Society guidelines; Ennis KJ, Reichard RA. Maximizing drug compliance in the elderly. Tips for staying on top of your patients' medication use. *Postgrad Med* 1997; 102: 211–24.

Box 2.5 **Evidence applied inappropriately to old people**

A 93-year-old lady with severe dementia is admitted to hospital from her nursing home with chest pain and non-specific changes on her electrocardiogram. Her performance status is poor. She is usually hoisted from bed to chair, is incontinent, and requires assistance for all activities of daily living. She is enrolled in the 'acute coronary syndrome protocol'. She is given aspirin 300 mg, clopidogrel 300 mg, simvastatin 40 mg and enoxaparin 50 mg twice daily by subcutaneous injection.

It is unclear whether the chest pain was angina, and if it was, whether it was stable angina or an acute coronary syndrome. No relevant trials have included patients of this age and co-morbidity. She is at higher risk of gastrointestinal bleeding compared to younger patients, may find regular injections distressing, and her long-term survival would not be affected by a statin.

---

reasons. Old patients are often excluded from clinical trials. Clinical application of evidence extrapolated from younger adults should sometimes be undertaken with caution. Interpreting evidence should be based on clinical significance as well as statistical significance, and the risks of adverse effects should be considered as well as the benefits. Box 2.5 shows an example of how 'evidence' is sometimes applied inappropriately to older people.

On the other hand, some drugs are under-prescribed in older people; for example, antidepressants, some treatments for heart failure, and warfarin. This is because of worries about side-effects despite evidence that the benefits outweigh the risks in this age group. Decision support tools (e.g. stroke risk for atrial fibrillation – see Chapter 7) or evidence-based resources may help in individual decision-making.

Better prescribing

How can prescribing in older patients be improved?

Box 2.6 **Drug-related problems that may be identified at a medication review**

- A medical condition is present that requires drug therapy but patient is not receiving any
- The patient has a medical condition for which the wrong drug is being taken
- Too little or too much of a correct drug is being taken
- The patient is suffering from an adverse drug reaction
- The patient has a problem resulting from a drug–drug, drug–food or drug–disease interaction
- The patient is taking a drug for which there is no valid indication

Review all medicines regularly

The Department of Health recommends that every person over the age of 75 has a medication review at least annually, the aim of which is to identify and resolve drug-related problems. Individual drugs and repeat prescriptions should be reviewed by the general practitioner or pharmacist. This has been shown to reduce the number of ADRs in older people. There is sometimes a reluctance to discontinue drugs if the patient has been on them for a long time, or if they were prescribed by another specialist. However, due to age-related changes, some drugs that were once beneficial may now be unnecessary or even causing harm. Box 2.6 outlines some drug-related problems that may be identified at a medication review.

Assess the patient

A good history, examination and any appropriate tests are important in making an accurate diagnosis. A drug history should include not just prescribed medication, but any 'borrowed' medication and over-the-counter drugs. Allergies should be clarified, as many patients are intolerant rather than truly allergic to drugs. Consideration should be given to the factors that affect compliance (listed in Box 2.3). Always consider that symptoms may be a side-effect of medication, in order to avoid a 'prescribing cascade' (Figure 2.3).

Think about non-pharmacological treatment

There are many non-pharmacological options available that should be considered first where appropriate, for example, dietary modification, physiotherapy or clinical psychology.

Think about the risks as well as the benefits

The appropriateness of a particular drug should be considered, taking into account the patient's perceptions, potential risks (side-effects, drug–drug and drug–disease interactions, the patient's physical status, and any compliance issues) versus potential benefits (quality of life and survival). Such risk vs benefit assessments may change over time in individual patients.

Start with a lower dose for most drugs

ADRs are closely related to the dose of drug. A 'start low and go slow' approach is often effective, with improved tolerability and compliance.

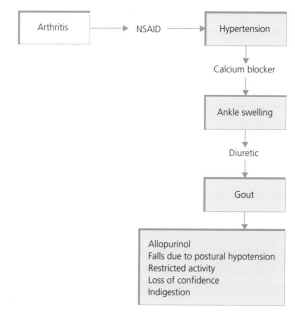

Figure 2.3 Prescribing cascade. Failure to recognise the side-effects of commonly prescribed drugs can lead to a 'prescribing cascade', resulting in unnecessary drug costs and reduced quality of life for an individual. A 78-year-old lady is prescribed a non-steroidal anti-inflammatory drug (NSAID) for arthritis of the knees. She then develops hypertension, a side-effect of this drug. She is put on a calcium blocker for hypertension, then develops ankle swelling, a side-effect of this drug. She is put on a diuretic for ankle swelling, then develops gout, a side-effect of this drug. She is put on allopurinol for gout, and then develops all the other complications listed: postural hypotension as a result of the calcium blocker and diuretic, leading to restricted activity and loss of confidence, and indigestion which is a side-effect of the NSAID.

Think about the route of administration

Some patients with poor dentition may find chewable tablets difficult to take. Some people may have swallowing problems, and others may have poor dexterity, making inhalers or pumped sprays difficult to use. In hospital or care homes it is especially important that certain regular medications are continued via a different route if the patient is temporarily unable to take them in the usual way. Examples include: anti-epileptic drugs, drugs for Parkinson's disease, angina medication, and long-term benzodiazepines.

Provide information and education

Adopting a patient-centred approach improves health outcomes for patients. Talking with patients about their disease and its treatment is an important part of concordance, particularly when starting a new drug or stopping old ones. Written information and involving relatives and carers (including care home staff), especially for people with cognitive impairment, is also helpful.

Further resources

Department of Health. (2001) *Medicines and older people: implementing medicines-related aspects of the NSF for Older People.* DH, London.

Fick DM, Cooper JW, Wade WE, Waller JL, Maclean JR, Beers MH. Medications to be avoided or used with caution in older patients. Updating the Beers criteria for potentially inappropriate medication use in older adults: results of a US consensus panel of experts. *Arch Intern Med* 2003; 163: 2716–24.

BMJ Clinical Evidence http://clinicalevidence.bmj.com

Acknowledgements

The authors would like to thank Dr Richard Fuller, Dr Sam Limaye and Dr Lauren Roulsten for their constructive comments on the manuscript.

CHAPTER 3

Delirium

John Holmes

OVERVIEW

- Delirium is common in older people, but is often not recognised
- It can present with a wide range of symptoms and signs
- Patients at high risk of developing delirium can be identified and it can sometimes be prevented
- Treatment of delirium involves environmental measures as well as treatment of the underlying cause
- Pharmacological treatment with sedatives or antipsychotic medication is a last resort

---

Delirium, or acute confusional state, is a common condition in older people. It frequently goes unrecognised and is often poorly managed. Patients who develop delirium have increased mortality, length of stay, complication and institutionalisation rates compared to non-delirious patients, independent of other factors. In up to one-third of cases, delirium can be prevented.

Aetiology

The aetiology of delirium is not fully understood. A genetic predisposition is possible. Inflammatory mediators may play a part. There is widespread cortical involvement in delirium, reflected in the wide range of symptoms, disturbances of conscious level and sleep–wake cycle, with illusions and hallucinations.

Although little is known of the pathophysiology of delirium, more is known about its predisposing and precipitating factors. These are shown in Box 3.1. Many of these factors occur commonly. If more predisposing factors are present, a lower severity of precipitating factor may provoke delirium.

Diagnosis

Delirium is particularly common in the post-operative period (43–61% after hip fracture, and higher in intensive care). It is also prevalent in the emergency department, affecting one in seven older patients. It is an acute condition, with symptoms developing over

---

Box 3.1 Predisposing and precipitating factors for delirium

Predisposing factors	Precipitating factors
Old age	Immobility
Severe illness	Use of physical restraint
Dementia	Use of urinary catheter
Physical frailty	Iatrogenic events e.g. general
Admission with infection or	anaesthesia
dehydration	Malnutrition
Visual/hearing impairment	Psychoactive medications
Polypharmacy	Intercurrent illness
Surgery e.g. fractured neck of femur	Dehydration
Alcohol excess	Benzodiazepine or alcohol
Renal impairment	withdrawal

From: Royal College of Physicians/British Geriatrics Society. (2006) *The prevention, diagnosis and management of delirium in older people. National guidelines.* RCP, London.

---

hours or days. People with delirium appear disorientated and are unable to focus their attention. Conversations are difficult to follow. Fluctuation in symptoms occurs, often with a diurnal pattern (i.e. worse at night), and lucid or symptom-free intervals may occur.

A diagnosis of delirium can be made when all four of the following features are present.

1. Acute onset.
2. Disturbance of consciousness.
3. Impaired cognition or perceptual disturbance, not due to pre-existing dementia.
4. Clinical evidence of an acute general medical condition, intoxication or substance withdrawal.

The International Classification of Diseases further describes the diagnostic features of delirium; these are outlined in Box 3.2. There are two main patterns of delirium:

- hyperactive delirium (agitated and wandering)
- hypoactive delirium (quiet and withdrawn).

Some patients may have features of both. The hypoactive pattern is particularly important because it often goes unrecognised. Affective symptoms are sometimes prominent in delirium and may lead to the erroneous diagnosis of a mood disorder. In patients with pre-existing dementia, delirium can be hard to spot. Delirium varies

ABC of Geriatric Medicine. Edited by N. Cooper, K. Forrest and G. Mulley. © 2009 Blackwell Publishing, ISBN: 978-1-4051-6942-4.

Box 3.2 **Diagnostic criteria for delirium**

Symptoms are present in the following areas:
1 **Disturbance of consciousness**
   - Reduced clarity of awareness of the environment, on a continuum from 'clouded consciousness' to coma, with a reduced ability to direct, focus, sustain and shift attention
2 **Global disturbance of cognition**
   - Perceptual distortions
   - Illusions and hallucinations – usually visual
   - Impaired abstract thinking and comprehension (with or without transient delusional beliefs)
   - Impaired immediate and recent memory but with relatively intact long-term memory
   - Disorientation in time, place or person
3 **Psychomotor disturbance**
   - Hyper- or hypoactivity and unpredictable shift from one to the other
   - Increased or decreased flow of speech
4 **Disturbance of the sleep–wake cycle**
   - Insomnia
   - Daytime drowsiness
   - Nocturnal worsening of symptoms
   - Disturbing dreams or nightmares
5 **Emotional disturbance**
   - Depression
   - Anxiety
   - Fear
   - Irritability
   - Euphoria
   - Apathy
   - Perplexity

(Acute alcohol and psychoactive substance use are excluded)

From: International Classification of Diseases (ICD) 10.

Box 3.3 **The Abbreviated Mental Test**

1 How old are you?
2 When is your birthday?
3 What time is it? (to the nearest hour)
4 Can you remember this address? 42 West Street
5 What year is it?
6 What place is this?
7 What is my job? What is that person's job? (Recognising two people)
8 Can you tell me the year World War One started or finished?
9 What is the name of the Monarch?
10 Can you count backwards from 20–1?

(Ask if the address 42 West Street is recalled at the end.)

This is a validated test; therefore asking any 10 of your own questions is not necessarily valid or reliable. Half-marks are not acceptable. A score of 8 or more is normal.

From: Hodgkinson HM. Evaluation of a mental test score for assessment of mental impairment in the elderly. *Age Ageing* 1972; 1: 233–8.

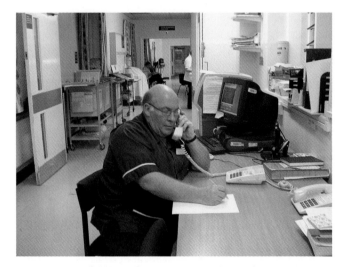

Figure 3.1 Get a full history from someone who knows the patient.

in both its severity and duration, and can last from a few days to several weeks.

National guidelines recommend that all older people should have routine cognitive testing on admission to hospital (e.g. using the Abbreviated Mental Test – see Box 3.3). This is to aid the detection of delirium.

The differential diagnosis of delirium includes:
- dementia
- depression
- hysteria
- mania
- schizophrenia
- dysphasia
- seizures (temporal lobe seizure or non-convulsive status epilepticus).

The most important aspect of diagnosis in delirium is to get a full history from someone who knows the patient (see Figure 3.1).

Management of delirium

Prevention
Those at high risk for developing delirium (see Box 3.1) can be targeted for proactive care aimed at preventing it. Some risk factors cannot be changed, but many in the list of precipitating factors can be. Other factors, including environmental ones, are also important in the prevention (and management) of delirium, and are listed in Box 3.4.

Detection
Half of all cases of delirium go unrecognised. Detection is more likely in those with difficult behaviours. Routine cognitive testing will not in itself identify delirium, but will alert the clinician to the presence of cognitive impairment and trigger further questions to differentiate delirium from dementia. Testing at presentation to acute medical services also gives a baseline for comparison later.

The Confusion Assessment Method (CAM) is designed to be used by any clinician (Box 3.5). Staff can be trained to use the screening instruments for detecting delirium, and these can be incorporated into routine care.

Box 3.4 **Other factors in the prevention and management of delirium**

Do the following:
- Ensure an appropriate environment:
  - avoid over-stimulation
  - ensure the patient is not deprived of spectacles and/or hearing aids
  - provide environmental and personal orientation
- Minimise discontinuity of care
- Encourage mobility
- Reduce medicines where possible (but ensure adequate analgesia)
- Maintain adequate fluid intake and nutrition
- Maintain normal sleep pattern
- Avoid constipation
- Involve relatives and carers
- Ensure regular medical, nursing and therapy reviews
- Avoid urinary catheters

Box 3.5 **Confusion Assessment Method (CAM)**

To have a positive CAM, the patient must display:
1 The presence of acute onset and fluctuating course
and
2 Inattention (e.g. counting from 20 to 1, with reduced ability to maintain or shift attention)
and either
3 (a) Disorganised thinking (disorganised or incoherent speech)
or
   (b) Altered level of consciousness (lethargic or stuporous)

Determining the underlying cause

When delirium has been detected, an assessment to look for the underlying cause is the next step. Several different acute illnesses, as well as medication, can produce delirium in at-risk patients. There is often more than one underlying cause. One in four patients will have at least two causes. Common causes of delirium are:
- infection (especially urine, chest and biliary)
- acute hypoxaemia
- electrolyte imbalance
- prescribed medicines
- myocardial infarction (which may be painless)
- alcohol or benzodiazepine withdrawal
- urinary retention
- faecal impaction
- neurological – stroke, subdural haematoma, seizures
- post-operative cognitive dysfunction (see Chapter 10).

The common drug groups that can cause delirium in older people are listed in Box 3.6.

The history, physical examination and inspection of the drug chart will often lead to the underlying cause. However, investigations are often needed and are shown in Box 3.7. First-line investigations are aimed at the more common causes of delirium. Second-line investigations should be requested in certain patients. Once the underlying causes have been identified, treatment should start without delay.

Box 3.6 **Common drug groups that can cause delirium in older people**

- Opioid analgesics
- Drugs with anticholinergic properties
- Sedating drugs e.g. benzodiazepines
- Corticosteroids

Box 3.7 **Investigations in delirium**

First-line investigations	Second-line investigations
Full blood count	Arterial blood gases
C-reactive protein	Computed tomography of the brain[*]
Urea and electrolytes	Electroencephalogram[†]
Calcium	Specific cultures e.g. wound swab,
Thyroid function tests	urine, sputum, blood or cerebrospinal
Liver function tests	fluid
Glucose	
Chest X-ray	
Electrocardiogram	
Pulse oximetry	
Urinalysis	

[*] If focal neurological signs, history of head injury or recurrent falls, evidence of raised intracranial pressure.
[†] If non-convulsive status epilepticus is suspected.

Treatment

People with delirium should be admitted to hospital, in order to facilitate observation, investigation and treatment. Treatment in delirium has four components:
1 treatment of the underlying cause(s)
2 environmental measures
3 pharmacological measures
4 prevention of complications.

There is good evidence that delirium incidence, severity and duration can be reduced through a multicomponent approach that ensures the delivery of good clinical care, focusing on the measures outlined in Box 3.4.

There are particular challenges in delivering even these simple interventions. For example, not all people in hospital can see a window or a clock, and the provision of a quiet, well-lit area to help avoid illusions may not be possible given the layout and facilities of many wards. Current hospital environments often make things worse. Patients may be moved between different wards, there is often constant activity and noise (see Figure 3.2) and a sea of unfamiliar faces, and there may be problems carrying out basic functions such as going to the toilet or eating. However, good holistic care from a multidisciplinary team can make a difference.

Staff who care for people with delirium should be adequately trained to manage the condition, which can include wandering, rambling speech and sometimes agitation and hallucinations. The least restrictive option should always be used. Distraction often works well. Communication should be optimised (e.g. by ensuring good lighting, spectacles and hearing aids) to find out the cause of any agitation. Relatives can be encouraged to stay with the patient. Arguing with, or restraining patients, usually makes things worse.

Pharmacological measures are a last resort and are indicated in the following situations.

• To prevent the patient endangering themselves or others.
• To allow essential investigations or treatment.
• To relieve distress in a highly agitated patient.

There is very little evidence on which drugs to use. Antipsychotics (e.g. haloperidol) are believed to treat the psychotic symptoms of delirium, but take several days to have an effect. In fact, the psychotic symptoms in delirium are treated by treating the underlying cause. Low doses of a short-acting benzodiazepine (e.g. lorazepam) are effective and possibly safer. The following two drugs are therefore recommended for use in delirium:

• lorazepam 0.5 mg orally
• haloperidol 0.5 mg orally.

Only one drug should be used, starting once a day in the evenings, and more frequently if necessary. In extreme agitation, larger doses may be given intramuscularly, under the supervision of an experienced doctor. If regular low doses do not work, there is little additional benefit (and an increase in side-effects), from giving more, and a mental health opinion should be sought. Further information on the use of these drugs in delirium can be found in *The Prevention, Diagnosis and Management of Delirium in Older People* in the further resources section at the end of this chapter.

The main complications of delirium are:

• falls
• pressure sores
• hospital-acquired infections
• functional impairment
• incontinence
• over-sedation
• malnutrition.

These should be actively prevented whenever possible and treated. Figure 3.3 summarises the prevention, diagnosis and management of a patient with delirium.

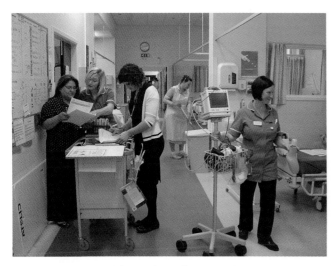

Figure 3.2 Constant activity on a busy admissions unit.

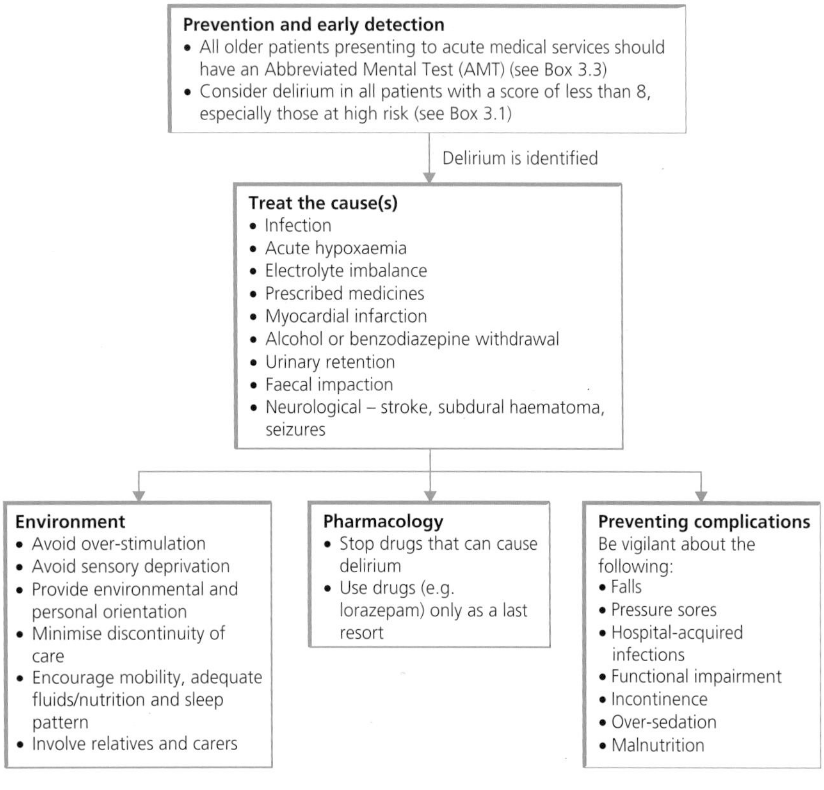

Prevention and early detection
• All older patients presenting to acute medical services should have an Abbreviated Mental Test (AMT) (see Box 3.3)
• Consider delirium in all patients with a score of less than 8, especially those at high risk (see Box 3.1)

Delirium is identified

Treat the cause(s)
• Infection
• Acute hypoxaemia
• Electrolyte imbalance
• Prescribed medicines
• Myocardial infarction
• Alcohol or benzodiazepine withdrawal
• Urinary retention
• Faecal impaction
• Neurological – stroke, subdural haematoma, seizures

Environment
• Avoid over-stimulation
• Avoid sensory deprivation
• Provide environmental and personal orientation
• Minimise discontinuity of care
• Encourage mobility, adequate fluids/nutrition and sleep pattern
• Involve relatives and carers

Pharmacology
• Stop drugs that can cause delirium
• Use drugs (e.g. lorazepam) only as a last resort

Preventing complications
Be vigilant about the following:
• Falls
• Pressure sores
• Hospital-acquired infections
• Functional impairment
• Incontinence
• Over-sedation
• Malnutrition

Figure 3.3 Summary of the prevention, diagnosis and management of delirium.

Challenges in delirium

Absence of an underlying cause

In up to a fifth of cases of delirium, an underlying cause cannot be found. In most, this is because delirium can persist long after the precipitating factor has resolved.

The aftermath

Patients who have had delirium may recall some or all of the events afterwards and be embarrassed or fearful. Research suggests that delirium is often a very unpleasant experience. An open and supportive approach can help. People who have had delirium are at increased risk of future episodes and this should be explained to them and their relatives and/or carers so that appropriate preventative action can be taken. The risk of developing dementia is increased after an episode, possibly due to delirium being a marker of reduced cerebral reserve, or a consequence of damage to the cerebral cortex by inflammatory mediators.

Difficult situations

The management of delirium may be hampered by lack of compliance from the patient. In severe cases, physical examination and investigations may be impossible. However, delirium is a medical emergency and its underlying cause should be treated as soon as possible. If patients lack mental capacity, they can be treated against their will, in their 'best interests' (which is legally defined – see further resources section in Chapter 15). Since delirium is a mental disorder, the Mental Health Act may also be used to detain patients, but is usually not necessary.

The future

Although delirium is common and detrimental, we still know little about its identification and management, which is frequently suboptimal. Acute medical services that cater for older people need to ensure that:

• high-risk patients are identified
• staff are trained to recognise and manage patients at risk of, or those who develop, delirium
• the environment is suitable for patients with delirium.

Further resources

Lindesay J, Rockwood K, Macdonald A, eds. (2002) *Delirium in Old Age*. Oxford University Press, Oxford.

Royal College of Physicians/British Geriatrics Society. (2006) *The prevention, diagnosis and management of delirium in older people. National guidelines*. RCP, London.

Royal College of Psychiatrists. (2005) *Who cares wins: improving the outcome for older people admitted to the general hospital. Report of a working group for the Faculty of Old Age Psychiatry*. RCPsych, London.

Siddiqi N, House AO, Holmes JD. Occurrence and outcome of delirium in medical inpatients: a systematic literature review. *Age Ageing* 2006; 35: 350–364.

Siddiqi N, Stockdale R, Britton AM, Holmes J. (2007) Interventions for preventing delirium in hospitalised patients. *Cochrane Database of Systematic Reviews* Issue 2, Art no: CD005563. DOI: 10.1002/14651858.CD005563. pub2.

CHAPTER 4

Falls

Nicola Cooper

OVERVIEW

- Falls in older people are common
- Recurrent falls are rarely 'mechanical' (i.e. accidental)
- The consequences of falls in older people include loss of confidence, loss of independence and fractures
- There is good evidence that simple interventions can prevent falls

Falls are a common presentation to GP surgeries, emergency departments and medical and orthopaedic admission units. The term 'mechanical' (i.e. accidental) fall is commonly used – accidental falls among older people admitted to hospital are uncommon, and recurrent falls should never be considered accidental. Older people often fall because of medical problems, many of which can be treated.

The problem of falls

For research purposes, the definition of a fall is 'unintentionally coming to rest on the ground or some lower level and other than as a consequence of sustaining a violent blow, loss of consciousness, or sudden onset of paralysis as in stroke or epileptic seizure'. Around one-third of people over the age of 65 living in their own homes fall each year. Half of all falls occur in the home, during routine activities of daily living, often with no obvious environmental hazard. The incidence of falls is higher for those living in institutions. Around half of care home residents who are mobile fall each year.

Falls in older people are more likely to lead to injuries. These occur in 50% of cases, mostly minor. In 1999 there were around 650 000 emergency department attendances for fall-related injuries in the over 60s. Even without an injury, some fallers are unable to get off the floor by themselves, which can lead to a 'long lie' causing dehydration, hypothermia, pressure sores and pneumonia. Falls also lead to loss of confidence and fear of falling. After a fall, half of older people report a fear of falls, and one-quarter limit their activities.

Around 5% of falls in older people lead to fractures. There are 86 000 hip fractures each year in the UK and 95% of these are the result of a fall. The total cost to the National Health Service is £1.7 billion per year – and this does not take into account loss of independence, reduced quality of life and costs to carers and social services.

Why do older people fall?

Falls in older people can be categorised into one of three groups:
- fall due to an acute illness
- single fall, which may be accidental
- recurrent falls.

A fall can be the presenting complaint for a range of acute illnesses in older people, and if faced with a person who has just fallen, you should screen for these (Box 4.1). The most common precipitating

---

Box 4.1 **Screening for acute illness in a patient who has just fallen**

History
- Of the fall itself (acute illness is more likely if new onset of frequent falls)
- Review of systems (e.g. symptoms of infection, new weakness)
- Medication review

Examination
- Of any injuries
- Vital signs, including respiratory rate
- Conjunctivae for severe anaemia
- Chest, abdomen and basic neurology (speech, visual fields, limbs)
- Lying and standing blood pressure (see Box 4.4)
- Watch the patient walk (see the 'get-up-and-go' test, Box 4.3)

Tests (depending on the facilities available)
- 12-lead ECG
- Urine dipstick
- Urea and electrolytes, glucose, C-reactive protein (CRP), full blood count

Remember that older patients may not have a raised white cell count or fever in sepsis (see Chapter 1), which is why the CRP is a useful test. Bacteruria in old ladies can be a normal finding and does not necessarily indicate urinary tract infection as the cause of a fall.

ABC of Geriatric Medicine. Edited by N. Cooper, K. Forrest and G. Mulley.
© 2009 Blackwell Publishing, ISBN: 978-1-4051-6942-4.

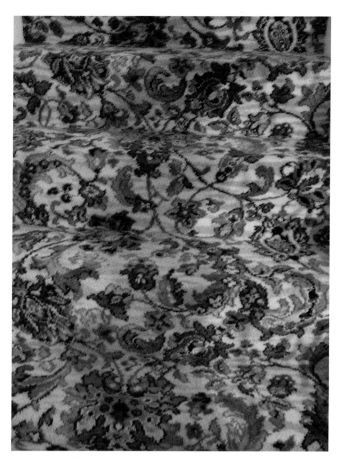

Figure 4.1 Stairs with a swirly patterned carpet. Ageing is associated with a decline in contrast sensitivity, or the ability to discriminate edges, accommodation and depth perception. About 10% of fall-related deaths occur on stairs and 75% of falls on stairs occur coming down, especially on the last step. Wearing bifocal or varifocal spectacles is an added risk factor for falls in this situation.

Box 4.2 **Risk factors for falls**

1 Social and demographic factors
- Advanced age
- Living alone
- Previous falls
- Limited activities of daily living

2 Age-related changes
- Reduced ability to discriminate edges (e.g. stairs)
- Reduced peripheral sensation
- Slower reaction times
- Muscle weakness

3 Poor gait and balance (postural instability)

4 Medical problems
- Cognitive impairment
- Parkinson's disease
- Cerebrovascular disease
- Eye diseases that reduce acuity (e.g. cataracts, glaucoma, age-related macular degeneration)
- Arthritis
- Foot problems
- Peripheral neuropathy
- Incontinence

5 Medications
- Psychiatric medication (e.g. antidepressants)
- Cardiovascular medication (e.g. antihypertensives)
- Being on four or more medications

6 Environmental factors
- Ill-fitting footwear (e.g. high heels, loose slippers)
- Wearing bifocal or varifocal spectacles

factor is infection, but others include haemorrhage, acute coronary syndromes and metabolic disturbances such as hyponatraemia and hyper- or hypoglycaemia.

Occasionally the clinician will come across a person who has had a genuine accidental fall (e.g. slipped on ice), who has a normal gait and balance and no other risk factors for falls. However, all older people presenting with a fall should have a basic falls assessment to look for any underlying cause (see later).

This chapter is mainly concerned with recurrent falls, i.e. people who have fallen more than once. Hundreds of different risk factors for recurrent falls have been identified, and are sometimes referred to as 'intrinsic' (e.g. muscle weakness, balance problems, poor vision, cognitive impairment) or 'extrinsic' (e.g. being on four or more prescription medications, environmental hazards – see Figure 4.1). Risk factors have a synergistic effect, so that risk rises dramatically as the number of risk factors increases. Risk factors for falls can be categorised into six main groups (Box 4.2).

There are particular risk factors for falls in institutions, and there is evidence that falls could be reduced if these are addressed (see Lord *et al.* in further resources section).

How to assess an older person who has fallen

The 2004 National Institute for Health and Clinical Excellence (NICE) guidelines on the assessment and prevention of falls in older people recommend that all people over the age of 65 in contact with a member of the healthcare team should be asked how many times they have fallen in the last 12 months. People reporting a fall, or deemed to be at risk of falls, should receive a basic assessment as they may benefit from participation in a local falls programme, which involves muscle strength and balance training, information and help (e.g. for home hazards).

Older people who require medical attention because of a fall or who report more than one fall in the last 12 months should receive a 'multifactorial falls risk assessment'. This is because recurrent falls usually have many causes (see Figure 4.2) and multifactorial interventions rather than single ones have been shown to be effective. A multifactorial assessment can be done by any trained member of the healthcare team, and usually involves more than one. The main components, *as well as* making any medical diagnoses, are vision assessment, medication modification, muscle strength and balance training, and assessment of home hazards. Home care staff and paramedics, as well as other healthcare professionals, should be able to refer people for such an assessment. Figure 4.3 summarises the basic and multifactorial risk assessments of an older person who has fallen. An action plan should follow.

Referral to a geriatrician with a special interest in falls is appropriate in the following situations:
- an abnormal gait and balance that require a diagnosis
- possible loss of consciousness
- when dizziness is a precipitating factor
- when medical conditions contributing to the falls could be optimised (e.g. postural hypotension, Parkinson's disease)

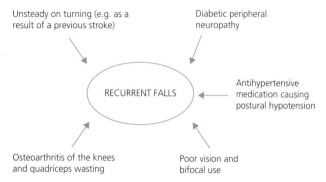

Figure 4.2 shows labelled around RECURRENT FALLS: Unsteady on turning (e.g. as a result of a previous stroke); Diabetic peripheral neuropathy; Antihypertensive medication causing postural hypotension; Osteoarthritis of the knees and quadriceps wasting; Poor vision and bifocal use.

Figure 4.2 Typical medical assessment of a patient with recurrent falls. Many of these problems can be improved by a combination of medical and physiotherapy interventions.

- recurrent unexplained falls (e.g. in patients with normal gait and balance).

Box 4.3 explains the 'get-up-and-go test' in more detail and Figure 4.4 outlines when admission to hospital is indicated after a fall.

The relationship between falls and syncope

Many older people are found lying on the floor without an eyewitness account of how they got there. It is impossible to decide whether a fall, syncope or seizure occurred – all are common in this age group. Cognitive impairment, retrograde amnesia or even a desire to explain the event means that older people often say they have tripped when they have not. Other causes (e.g. syncope) should be considered as a cause of falls when the falls are unexplained or the patient cannot remember hitting the ground.

In the SAFE PACE study, older people attending an emergency department because of falls without loss of consciousness were screened for carotid sinus hypersensitivity, a condition that causes transient bradycardia and hypotension when the carotid body in the neck is pressed or stretched. Of those who were diagnosed as having

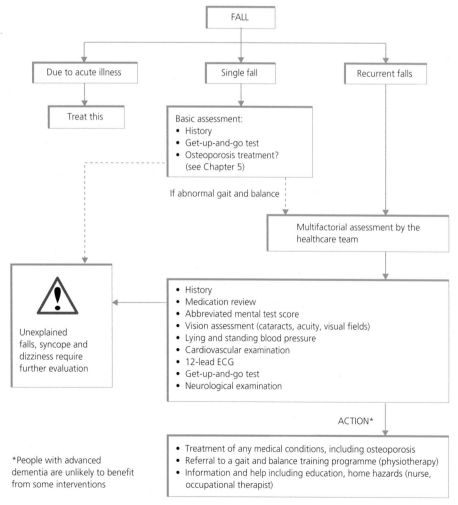

Figure 4.3 Assessment of an older person who has fallen.

*People with advanced dementia are unlikely to benefit from some interventions

Box 4.3 **The get-up-and-go test**

The get-up-and-go test is a simple screening test for gait and balance abnormalities. The patient is asked to rise from a chair (without using his or her arms if possible), walk 3 metres, turn around, return to the chair and sit down again.

Typical diagnoses that can be suspected by watching a patient walk include:
- previous stroke
- peripheral neuropathy
- Parkinsonism
- severe arthritis
- cerebellar or vestibular problems
- foot drop.

An abnormal gait and balance should be further investigated by a neurological examination. For example, cord compression due to degenerative changes of the spine is not an uncommon finding in a specialist falls clinic.

A lot of useful information can still be gained by walking with a patient who needs assistance for a short distance.

Box 4.4 **Postural (orthostatic) hypotension**

For diagnostic purposes, the patient should lie supine for 5 minutes and have their blood pressure measured lying, immediately after standing, and after 3 minutes of standing.

Postural hypotension is present when the systolic blood pressure falls by more than 20 mmHg, or the diastolic blood pressure by more than 10 mmHg.

The patient may or may not have symptoms.

Older patients with recurrent unexplained falls should be considered for syncope investigations, for example, tilt testing and carotid sinus massage. Carotid sinus massage should ideally be performed in a tilt test room both supine and upright. It is a safe test, with a less than 1% risk of neurological complications. Further information is given in Chapter 6.

Dizziness and falls

Dizziness is frequently associated with falls and is a common symptom in older people. There are three patterns of dizziness:
- light-headedness or 'not right' on standing or walking around
- vertigo
- 'fuzzy all the time'.

Light-headed episodes independent of posture can be caused by hypoglycaemia or cardiac arrhythmias and will not be considered further. Postural (orthostatic) hypotension is common in older people (see Box 4.4), but many do not describe their symptoms as 'light-headedness', instead referring to feeling 'not right' or 'off balance' when standing or walking. If the symptoms are mainly present when upright or walking around, postural hypotension should be suspected, particularly if the individual tends to have a low blood pressure or is taking antihypertensive medication. Many older people have a blood pressure that falls slowly after assuming the upright position, and a simple lying and standing blood pressure may not detect any change. A tilt test can be used to investigate this further in the context of collapses (see Chapter 6).

Vertigo refers to a sensation of movement in any direction and does not necessarily mean 'spinning'. Four main types of vertigo are outlined in Figure 4.5. Benign paroxysmal positional vertigo (BPPV) is extremely common and can present with balance problems and falls in older people as well as the classical brief vertigo on looking up. Posterior canal BPPV is the most common type and is diagnosed by the Dix–Hallpike manoeuvre and treated by the Epley manoeuvre (see Figure 4.6). The other types of vertigo shown can also be successfully treated (see Furman and Cass in further resources section).

Brief vertigo on looking up is often attributed to vertebrobasilar insufficiency, which is rare and does not cause vertigo alone; or cervical spondylosis, which is a common X-ray finding but is controversial as a cause of dizziness, does not cause vertigo alone, and should not be considered an adequate explanation.

'Fuzzy all the time' is a particularly frustrating form of dizziness, and in older people may be associated with diffuse cerebrovascular

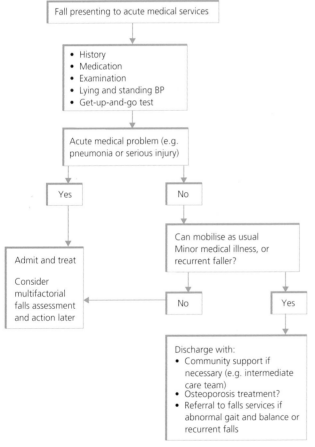

Figure 4.4 When admission to hospital is required following a fall.

cardioinhibitory carotid sinus hypersensitivity (the most common type, which causes bradycardia), half were randomised to receive a dual chamber pacemaker and half to receive usual falls care. There was a two-thirds reduction in falls in the paced group, suggesting an association between falls and carotid sinus hypersensitivity.

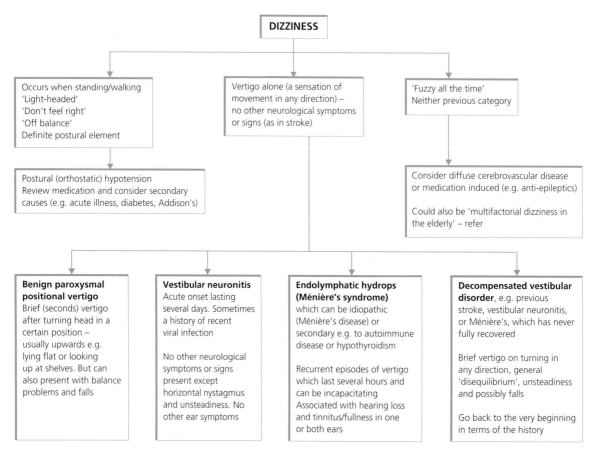

Figure 4.5 Patterns of dizziness in older people. An additional cause of vertigo alone is migrainous vertigo, more common in younger people. This can present with attacks of vertigo lasting up to one hour, with or without headache, or with symptoms of a decompensated vestibular disorder, or both.

disease or medication. Sometimes it is compounded by other things that cause dizziness (e.g. postural hypotension or a vestibular problem) and in addition the patient may have poor vision/bifocals and a peripheral neuropathy. This syndrome is referred to as 'multifactorial dizziness in the elderly' [sic]. As well as having more than one type of dizziness, there are multiple pathologies in different parts of the body that together produce a sensation of disequilibrium most of the time. These patients can be helped by referral to a geriatric team with a special interest in dizziness.

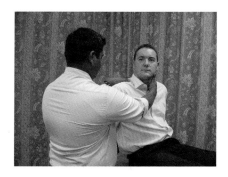

1 To test the right ear, the patient sits on a couch with the head turned to the right

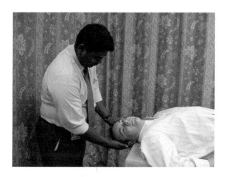

2 The clinician supports the neck, as the patient lies flat as quickly as possible, with the head slightly dangling over the edge of the couch so that the chin points slightly upwards, still turned to the right. This may produce vertigo and nystagmus. The hallmarks of nystagmus in posterior canal BPPV are delayed (by up to 20 seconds), rotational (towards the affected side), and fatigueable (it gets less each time the manoeuvre is performed)

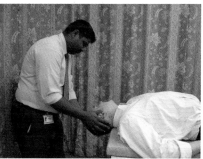

3 The vertigo and nystagmus settle after a few minutes, then the patient's head is turned to the opposite side

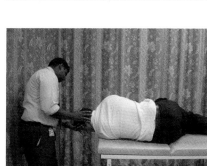

4 After a further few minutes, the patient's head is turned to look down at the floor. He has to turn on his side to do this

Figure 4.6 The Hallpike and Epley manoeuvres for BPPV. Most benign paroxysmal positional vertigo (BPPV) is caused by a problem with the posterior semicircular canal in the inner ear. It is diagnosed on the basis of history, normal neurological examination and a positive Dix–Hallpike manoeuvre (pictures 1 and 2) which produces transient vertigo and *characteristic* nystagmus. If positive, the clinician can go on to perform the Epley manoeuvre (pictures 3, 4 and 5), which repositions stray endolymphatic debris which is the cause of the symptoms. In 75% of cases of BPPV, symptoms spontaneously resolve in a month or two. But for those whose symptoms persist, the Epley manoeuvre is extremely effective and can be performed with assistance even in frail elderly patients. For a more detailed explanation, see Furman and Cass in further resources section.

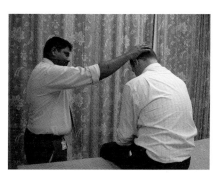

5 After a further few minutes, and with the head still turned towards the left shoulder, the patient is assisted into a sitting position. Once upright, the head is tilted so that the chin points slightly downward

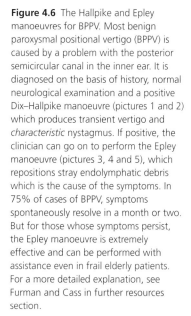

Further resources

National Institute for Health and Clinical Excellence. (2004) Falls. The assessment and prevention of falls in older people. *Clinical Guideline 21.* www.nice.org.uk

Lord SR, Sherrington S, Menz HB. (2001) *Falls in Older People – Risk Factors and Strategies for Prevention.* Cambridge University Press.

American Geriatrics Society, British Geriatrics Society and American Academy of Orthopaedic Surgeons panel on falls prevention. Guidelines for the prevention of falls in older persons. *J Am Geriatr Soc* 2001; 49(5): 664–72.

Kenny RA, Richardson DA, Steen N *et al.* Carotid sinus syndrome: a modifiable risk factor for non-accidental falls in older adults (SAFE PACE). *J Am Coll Cardiol* 2001; 38(5): 1491–6.

Furman JM, Cass SP. (2003) *Vestibular Disorders. A Case-study Approach*, 2nd edn. Oxford University Press.

CHAPTER 5

Bone Health

Katrina Topp

OVERVIEW

- Maintenance of bone health is important to prevent debilitating fractures
- Osteoporosis is the most common cause of fragility fractures in older people
- Vitamin D deficiency and insufficiency are also common in older people and contribute to falls and fractures
- Lifestyle advice should be given to promote and improve bone health
- Calcium, vitamin D and bisphosphonates are first-line therapy for osteoporosis but other medications are also available

The promotion and maintenance of bone health in older people is vitally important in order to reduce the incidence of fragility fractures related to falls. A fragility fracture is defined as a fracture sustained when falling from standing height or less. Falls are a major cause of disability and the leading cause of mortality due to injury in people aged over 75 in the UK (see Chapter 4). Osteoporosis increases the risk of fracture when a person falls, and up to 14 000 people each year in the UK die as a result of an osteoporotic hip fracture.

The National Institute for Health and Clinical Excellence (NICE), Royal College of Physicians and the National Osteoporosis Society have issued guidance on bone health which recommends lifestyle changes, good nutrition and pharmacological treatment for those at risk of osteoporosis and vitamin D deficiency.

Osteoporosis

Osteoporosis is defined by the World Health Organization (WHO) as 'a progressive, systemic skeletal disease characterised by low bone mass and micro-architectural deterioration of bone tissue, with a consequent increase in bone fragility and susceptibility to fracture.' Often known as 'the silent disease', due to the slowly progressive and asymptomatic decline of skeletal tissue, there may be no clinical signs until a person presents with a painful fracture. The most common areas for fracture are the spine (Figure 5.1), wrist and hip

ABC of Geriatric Medicine. Edited by N. Cooper, K. Forrest and G. Mulley.
© 2009 Blackwell Publishing, ISBN: 978-1-4051-6942-4.

(Figure 5.2); but the general nature of the condition means that any bone may be involved. Chronic pain, disability, loss of independence and premature death may result, which is why it is important to identify and manage those at risk.

Aetiology

Osteoporosis predominantly affects post-menopausal women as a result of oestrogen deficiency but it also occurs in men. One in three women and one in twelve men will suffer an osteoporotic fracture after the age of 50. The incidence of osteoporosis rises with increasing age but fracture risk is higher in older people compared with younger people with the same bone mineral density. Around half of cases in men are associated with hypogonadism (20%), corticosteroid use (20%) or alcohol excess (5%) so these risk factors should be specifically sought. Secondary causes of osteoporosis (see Box 5.1) occur in both sexes.

Diagnosis

The standard for the diagnosis of osteoporosis is assessment of bone mineral density (BMD) by axial dual-energy X-ray absorptiometry (DEXA). A diagnosis of osteoporosis may also be suspected from any of the following:
- marked osteopenia on plain X-ray
- a previous fragility fracture
- the identification of risk factors for osteoporosis.

The WHO classification of osteoporosis has been widely adopted and is based on the measurement of BMD with reference to the number of standard deviations (SD) from the mean in an average 25-year-old woman, known as the T-score (see Box 5.2). The threshold for osteoporosis is at least 2.5 SD below this reference point (i.e. a T-score of −2.5 or more). T-scores can vary by anatomical site so the prediction of fracture risk is usually based on measurements estimated at the femoral neck as this is most predictive of hip fracture (the major cause of loss of independence, mortality and cost).

Assessing fracture risk

Although low BMD is helpful in assessing fracture risk, it does not alone predict whether a person will sustain a fracture in absolute

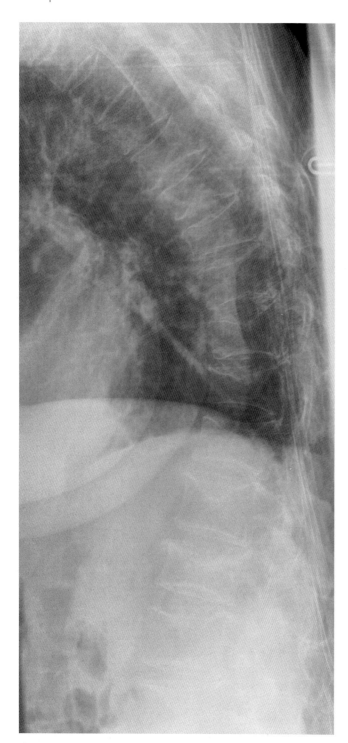

Figure 5.1 Lateral thoracic spine X-ray showing osteopenia and multiple wedge vertebral collapses.

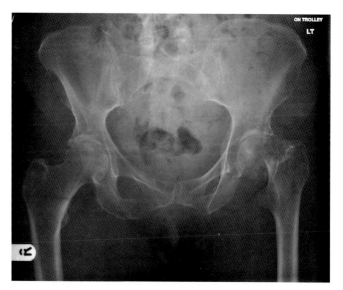

Figure 5.2 Pelvic X-ray showing osteopenia and a displaced subcapital fracture of the left neck of femur.

Box 5.1 **Risk factors for the development of osteoporosis**

Non-modifiable
- Female gender
- Family history of osteoporosis (especially maternal history of hip fracture at less than 75 years old)
- Caucasian or Asian ethnicity
- Age more than 65 years
- Previous fragility fracture

Modifiable
- Low body mass index (less than 19 kg/m^2)
- Smoking
- Alcohol excess
- Low calcium intake and vitamin D deficiency
- Inactivity

Hormonal
- Menopause before age 45 years or prolonged untreated amenorrhoea
- Male hypogonadism

Secondary causes
- Rheumatoid arthritis
- Hyperthyroidism
- Malabsorption (particularly coeliac disease)
- Chronic liver disease
- Primary hyperparathyroidism
- Prolonged immobilisation
- Anorexia nervosa

Drugs
- Glucocorticoids
- Anticonvulsants
- Prolonged heparin therapy
- Cytotoxic therapy

terms. Other factors such as a tendency to fall should also be considered. Those who have already had one fragility fracture are at highest risk of sustaining further fractures and should be prioritised for investigation and treatment. Over the past few years many meta-analyses have been carried out to identify risk factors that could be used to identify those at risk of osteoporosis and fracture. A 10-year fracture prediction tool, currently in development,

incorporates clinical risk factors that are independent of BMD. These include:
- age
- prior fragility fracture
- smoking history
- excess alcohol use
- a family history of hip fracture
- rheumatoid arthritis
- systemic corticosteroid use.

Investigations in osteoporosis or after a fragility fracture

Patients with osteoporosis and/or a fragility fracture will need further investigation to exclude secondary causes of the disease and other causes of a pathological fracture. These are outlined in Box 5.3.

The role of vitamin D

Vitamin D regulates calcium and phosphate absorption and metabolism, and is essential for bone health. Our main source of vitamin D is through the action of sunlight on the skin to produce vitamin D3 and a smaller contribution is made from diet (e.g. vitamin D2 from vegetables or D3 from meat). These metabolites are converted initially in the liver and then in the kidneys to the fully active metabolite 1,25-dihydroxycholecalciferol. Primary vitamin D deficiency is more common in individuals who have little exposure to the sun as well as those with an inadequate diet. It is common in older people, and is found in at least a third of those aged over 65 years. Lesser degrees of vitamin D deficiency may be found in as many as 55% of this age group. Symptoms may range from none at all, through to insidious onset of muscular and bony aches and pains, to frank osteomalacia. In the presence of osteoporosis, vitamin D deficiency exacerbates bone loss and can provoke secondary hyperparathyroidism which substantially increases the risk of fractures.

Treatment for osteoporosis

Lifestyle changes

Patients should be advised to stop smoking and reduce alcohol consumption if this is excessive. It is important to promote a healthy balanced diet with good calcium intake (see Box 5.4) and to maintain vitamin D levels through diet and appropriate sun exposure (suberythemal exposure to the face, arms, hands or back for 15 minutes, two or three times a week). A high salt intake may also increase bone loss. Use of oral corticosteroids should be kept to a minimum and consideration given to steroid-sparing agents if required long term. A Cochrane systematic review has shown

Box 5.4 **Calcium content of foods**

Food	Milligrams of calcium/100 g of food
Daily products	
Edman cheese	795
Cheddar cheese	739
Semi-skimmed milk (100 mL)	120
Fish	
Whitebait, fried	860
Sardines in oil	500
Sardines in tomato sauce	250
Salmon, tinned	91
Tuna, tinned in oil	12
Vegetables	
Okra, stir fried	220
Spinach boiled	160
Watercress	170
Pulses, beans and seeds	
Sesame seeds	670
Red kidney beans	71
Green/French beans	56
Cereal products	
Ready Brek	1200
White bread	177
Wholemeal bread	106
Fruit	
Figs, dried	250
Orange	47

Adapted from National Osteoporosis Society patient information leaflet *Calcium Rich Foods*.

that regular weight-bearing exercise is effective in preventing and treating osteoporosis in post-menopausal women.

Pharmacological treatments

Calcium and vitamin D

Daily supplementation with calcium (1200 mg) and vitamin D (800 IU) should be offered to all institutionalised older people as this is proven to reduce fractures in a meta-analysis of randomised controlled trials (RCTs) and a Cochrane systematic review. NICE recommends that all patients treated for osteoporosis with other therapies should also receive calcium and vitamin D supplementation unless the clinician is confident that levels are normal, or there are contraindications (e.g. hypercalcaemia).

Bisphosphonates

Bisphosphonates act by reducing the rate of bone turnover and have an important role in both the prevention and treatment of osteoporosis. Three bisphosphonates, alendronate, risedronate and cyclic etidronate, are specifically licensed for the prevention and treatment of post-menopausal and glucocorticoid-induced osteoporosis, but only alendronate is licensed for use in men.

Alendronate and risedronate can be given daily or weekly. They have been proven in RCTs to produce statistically significant reductions in the incidence of vertebral, non-vertebral and hip fractures. Alendronate can cause oesophagitis and is contraindicated when a patient has abnormalities of the oesophagus that delay emptying (e.g. stricture or achalasia), but risedronate may be used with caution. Both should be avoided if renal function is impaired (a glomerular filtration rate (GFR) of less than 35 mL/min).

Cyclical etidronate is given daily in a cycle with calcium carbonate. It is effective in reduction of vertebral fractures but has not been proven in pooled RCTs to reduce non-vertebral or hip fractures. It has few upper gastrointestinal side-effects. It is contraindicated in moderate to severe renal impairment.

Raloxifene

Raloxifene is a selective oestrogen receptor modulator and is licensed for the prevention and treatment of vertebral fractures in post-menopausal women. Its most serious side-effect is a threefold increase in the risk of venous thromboembolism. It can also cause hypertension.

Strontium ranelate

Strontium ranelate has a dual action of stimulating new bone formation and reducing bone resorption. It is licensed for the treatment of post-menopausal osteoporosis and is proven in RCTs to reduce the incidence of both vertebral and hip fractures. There may be a small increase in the risk of venous thromboembolism. It should also be avoided in renal impairment (a GFR of less than 30 mL/min).

Teriparatide

Teriparatide is a recombinant fragment of parathyroid hormone given as a daily subcutaneous injection for 18 months. It is licensed for the treatment of post-menopausal osteoporosis and reduces

---

Box 5.5 NICE guidance for the secondary prevention of osteoporotic fragility fractures in post-menopausal women

Calcium and/or vitamin D supplementation should be provided to those who receive osteoporosis treatment if it is suspected that levels are inadequate.

Treatment groups
- Aged 75 years and older – DEXA scan not required
- Aged 65–74 years – DEXA scan confirms osteoporosis (T-score <−2.5)
- Younger than 65 years – DEXA scan confirms osteoporosis with
  - T-score <−3 or
  - T-score <−2.5 PLUS one or more age-independent risk factors:
    - body mass index <19 kg/m^2
    - maternal hip fracture before age 75 years
    - untreated premature menopause
    - medical disorders associated with bone loss (e.g. hyperthyroidism)
    - conditions associated with prolonged immobility.

Treatment guidance
- Bisphosphonates (alendronate, etidronate and risedronate) are recommended as first-line therapy.
- Raloxifene as second-line therapy if:
  - bisphosphonates are contraindicated or patient is unable to comply with recommendations for use
  - an unsatisfactory response to bisphosphonates
  - intolerant of bisphosphonates.
- Teriparatide as second-line therapy in those aged 65 years and older if:
  - unsatisfactory response or intolerance to bisphosphonates and
  - T-score <−4 or
  - T-score <−3 PLUS >2 fractures PLUS one or more age-independent risk factors:
    - body mass index <19 kg/m^2
    - maternal hip fracture before age 75 years
    - untreated premature menopause
    - medical disorders associated with bone loss (e.g. hyperthyroidism)
    - conditions associated with prolonged immobility.

Unsatisfactory response is defined as a further fragility fracture despite adhering to treatment for 1 year plus evidence of decline in baseline BMD. Intolerance of bisphosphonates is defined as oesophageal ulceration, erosion or stricture, or severe lower gastrointestinal symptoms.

---

vertebral and non-vertebral fractures. It should be initiated only by a secondary care specialist in osteoporosis.

Calcitonin

Parenteral calcitonin is licensed for the treatment of post-menopausal osteoporosis. A systematic review has shown a reduction in vertebral and non-vertebral fractures but to a lesser extent than bisphosphonates.

Hormone replacement therapy (HRT)

Although HRT has been shown to reduce vertebral and non-vertebral fractures, it is no longer recommended for long-term use

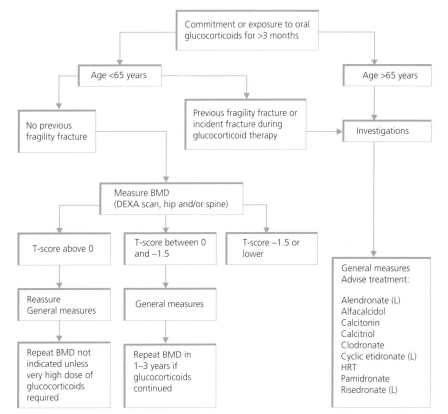

Figure 5.3 Management of glucocorticoid-induced osteoporosis in men and women (taken from the Royal College of Physicians, Bone and Tooth Society of Great Britain and National Osteoporosis Society guidelines. See further resources section). BMD, bone mineral density; DEXA, dual-energy X-ray absorptiometry; (L), licensed for glucocorticoid-induced osteoporosis. A fragility fracture is defined as a fracture occurring on minimal trauma after age 40 years and includes forearm, spine, hip, ribs and spine. General measures include:

- Reduce dose of glucocorticoid when possible
- Consider glucocorticoid-sparing therapy if possible
- Recommend good nutrition, especially with adequate calcium and vitamin D
- Recommend regular weight-bearing exercise
- Maintain body weight
- Avoid tobacco use and alcohol abuse
- Assess falls risk and give advice if appropriate

because of an increased risk of breast cancer and cardiovascular disease.

National osteoporosis guidelines

NICE issued guidance on the secondary prevention of osteoporotic fragility fractures in post-menopausal women in January 2005 (see Box 5.5). This did not include strontium ranelate, but an updated guideline is currently being produced. NICE guidance on the primary prevention of post-menopausal osteoporotic fragility fractures is also in development. The treatment and prevention of glucocorticoid-induced osteoporosis was excluded by NICE; however, the Royal College of Physicians issued guidance on this in 2002, which is outlined in Figure 5.3.

Further resources

National Institute for Health and Clinical Excellence. (2005) Bisphosphonates (alendronate, etidronate and risedronate), selective oestrogen receptor modulators (raloxifene) and parathyroid hormone (teriparatide) for the secondary prevention of osteoporotic fragility fractures in post-menopausal women. *Technology Appraisal 87*. NICE, London. www.nice.org.uk

Royal College of Physicians and Bone and Tooth Society of Great Britain. (2000) Osteoporosis: clinical guidelines for prevention and treatment. Update on pharmacological interventions and an algorithm for management. Royal College of Physicians, London. www.rcplondon.ac.uk

Royal College of Physicians, Bone and Tooth Society of Great Britain and National Osteoporosis Society. (2002) Glucocorticoid-induced osteoporosis: guidelines for prevention and treatment. Royal College of Physicians, London. www.rcplondon.ac.uk

Primary vitamin D deficiency in adults. *Drugs Therapeut Bull* 2006; 44: 25–28.

The National Osteoporosis Society. www.nos.org.uk

CHAPTER 6

Syncope

Raja Hussain

OVERVIEW

- Collapse with transient loss of consciousness is a common clinical problem
- The most important diagnostic tool is the history, including an eye-witness account if possible
- In syncope, the underlying cause will be obvious in more than one-third of cases after history, examination, lying and standing blood pressure and a 12-lead electrocardiogram
- Unexplained syncope requires investigation if it is recurrent, or if a single episode led to a significant injury
- People with structural heart disease require cardiac investigations for syncope

'Collapse' usually refers to an episode of transient loss of consciousness leading to a fall. In clinical practice, the main differential diagnosis when a person collapses or has a 'blackout' is syncope or a seizure.

An overview of syncope

The word 'syncope' is derived from the Greek 'syn' (with) and 'koptein' (to interrupt). It is characterised by transient, self-limiting loss of consciousness, usually leading to a fall. The onset is relatively rapid and recovery is spontaneous, complete and *usually* prompt. Syncope is always the result of transient global cerebral hypoperfusion, and there are different causes.

Syncope accounts for up to 5% of emergency department visits, and can have a major impact on lifestyle. In older people its prevalence is higher, injuries and loss of confidence are more common, and so is admission to hospital. Isolated episodes are common. If a person has experienced more than one episode, it is more likely to recur. The prevalence of syncope in older people may be underestimated because it can also present as 'falls' because of retrograde amnesia or lack of eye witnesses.

Older people are at higher risk of syncope because of age-related physiological changes in heart rate, blood pressure, cerebral

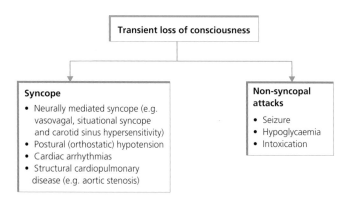

Figure 6.1 The different causes of transient loss of consciousness. A transient ischaemic attack (TIA) causes loss of focal neurology rather than loss of consciousness. Posterior circulation TIAs can cause transient loss of consciousness, but this is in addition to other neurological symptoms and signs.

blood flow, baroreceptor sensitivity and blood volume regulation. In addition, they have a high prevalence of diseases that can predispose to syncope and are often taking several prescribed medications.

Figure 6.1 shows the main causes of collapse, divided into syncope and non-syncopal attacks. The four main categories of syncope are also shown.

Neurally mediated syncope refers to vasovagal syncope (fainting) and situational syncope (e.g. micturition syncope). A neurally mediated reflex is triggered, leading to vasodilation and bradycardia (vagal stimulation), causing hypotension and cerebral hypoperfusion. Carotid sinus hypersensitivity is also neurally mediated. In this case the reflex is triggered by pressure on the carotid body.

Postural (orthostatic) hypotension is the result of impaired autonomic reflexes, leading to pooling of blood in the veins of the lower limbs. Volume depletion is another cause.

Tachy- or bradycardias can reduce cardiac output, leading to cerebral hypoperfusion and syncope. Structural cardiopulmonary disease can also lead to syncope when there is an impaired ability to increase cardiac output (e.g. in aortic stenosis or hypertrophic obstructive cardiomyopathy). Figure 6.2 outlines the main categories of syncope in more detail.

ABC of Geriatric Medicine. Edited by N. Cooper, K. Forrest and G. Mulley.
© 2009 Blackwell Publishing, ISBN: 978-1-4051-6942-4.

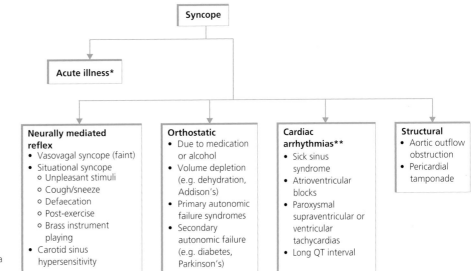

Figure 6.2 The main causes of syncope.

*A range of acute illnesses can cause syncope, including infection, dehydration, acute cardiac ischaemia, haemorrhage, aortic dissection and pulmonary embolism.
**A normal electrocardiogram virtually excludes a cardiac cause of syncope.

In older people, the most common causes of syncope are:
- postural hypotension (20–30%)
- carotid sinus hypersensitivity (20%)
- cardiac arrhythmias (20%)
- vasovagal or situational syncope (15%).

This is different to young people in whom vasovagal and situational syncope are far more common and carotid sinus hypersensitivity is extremely rare.

How to assess a patient with a collapse

A thorough history is essential in the evaluation of any collapse. A detailed account of the incident from the patient, *and any available eye witnesses* (over the telephone if necessary) is crucial. Past medical history, medications, cardiovascular and neurological examination, lying and standing blood pressure and 12-lead electrocardiogram are the other essential components of the evaluation. Patients should also be asked about their social circumstances and whether or not they drive. Box 6.1 outlines the key questions that should be asked in the history. Syncope is characterised by a brief loss of consciousness, with few abnormal movements, pallor and a quick recovery. Box 6.2 outlines the main differences between syncope and seizures.

If the history suggests syncope (as opposed to a seizure or other non-syncopal attack), the key questions are as follows.

1 Is there an acute illness? (Syncope can be the presenting feature in a wide range of acute illnesses e.g. sepsis, bleeding.)
2 If no acute illness, is the cause of syncope obvious after the initial evaluation?
3 Does the patient have structural heart disease?
4 Does the patient drive?

After a full history, examination, lying and standing blood pressure and 12-lead electrocardiogram, the cause of syncope will be apparent in at least one-third of cases. For example, syncope due to postural hypotension as a result of medication is common in older people. This can be diagnosed and treated without further tests.

Box 6.1 Key questions in the history

Questions about before the attack
- Position (lying, sitting or standing)
- Activity (e.g. change in posture, during or after exercise, micturition)
- Predisposing factors (e.g. warm environment, prolonged standing)
- Precipitating factors (e.g. unpleasant stimuli, concurrent illness, *chest pain, neck movements*)
- Prodromal symptoms (e.g. feeling warm, nauseated, blurred vision)

The four Ps are strongly suggestive of vasovagal syncope: upright *position*, *predisposing* factors, certain *precipitating* factors (those not in italics) and a typical *prodrome*.

Questions about during the attack (from an eye witness)
- How the person fell (floppy or rigid)
- What colour they were (white or blue)
- Whether they were allowed to lie flat or someone held them upright
- The presence of any tonic-clonic movements and their duration
- Any injuries or incontinence

Questions about after the attack
- What the person was like when they came round
- How long it took to recover

Background questions
- History of cardiac disease
- Past medical history
- Medications
- History of previous collapses and their circumstances
- Whether or not the person had a tendency to faint when younger
- Whether or not they go dizzy on standing quickly or after standing for a long time

Patients with structural heart disease and syncope have a higher mortality (see Box 6.3). A person is considered to have structural heart disease if they have one of the following: a history of heart disease (e.g. previous myocardial infarction, heart failure), a clinically significant murmur (e.g. aortic stenosis), or an abnormal

Box 6.2 **The main differences between syncope and seizures**

The overall picture is more important than any single feature.

Syncope more likely	Seizure more likely
Upright posture	Aura (e.g. funny smell)
Pallor, nausea/vomiting, sweaty, warm	Cyanosis
Brief jerking movements may occur after the patient has lost consciousness	Prolonged tonic-clonic movements or rigidity that coincides with loss of consciousness
	Automatisms, tongue biting
Quick recovery (if allowed to lie flat)	Prolonged confusion, headache or drowsiness*
Fatigue afterwards is common	At night in bed
Incontinence of urine can occur	Faecal incontinence

*If a person sustains a head injury during syncope, these features may be present due to concussion.

Box 6.3 **Prognosis in recurrent syncope**

Poor prognosis
- Structural heart disease (independent of the cause of syncope)

Excellent prognosis
- Young, healthy patient with normal electrocardiogram
- Neurally mediated reflex syncope
- Orthostatic hypotension
- Unexplained syncope after thorough evaluation (around 20% of cases)

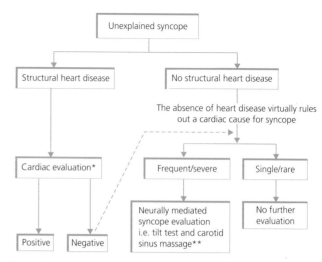

Figure 6.3 Summary of the European Society of Cardiology guidelines on the investigation of unexplained syncope. Structural heart disease = previous myocardial infarction, clinically significant murmur (e.g. aortic stenosis), abnormal electrocardiogram. (In young people a family history of sudden cardiac death is also included.)

*Troponin is not indicated in syncope without chest pain or acute electrocardiogram abnormalities. Cardiac evaluation may include 24-hour electrocardiogram or more prolonged monitoring, echocardiogram, electrophysiology studies in selected patients, implantable loop recorder in selected patients.

**Carotid sinus massage is indicated only in people over the age of 50 years. Contraindications to carotid sinus massage include recent stroke or TIA, significant carotid artery stenosis, history of ventricular tachyarrhythmias, recent myocardial infarction.

electrocardiogram. An abnormal electrocardiogram refers to atrial fibrillation or flutter, atrioventricular blocks, previous myocardial infarction or an abnormal QT interval, rather than non-specific ST changes.

If the cause of syncope is unclear after the initial evaluation, patients with structural heart disease require cardiac investigations. Patients without structural heart disease require different tests (e.g. tilt test and/or carotid sinus massage). Figure 6.3 shows a flow chart based on the European Society of Cardiology guidelines on the investigation of *unexplained* syncope.

All patients should be asked whether or not they drive. For vasovagal syncope and postural hypotension, there are no driving restrictions in UK law. The Driver and Vehicle Licensing Authority (DVLA) website has up-to-date information on driving regulations for doctors. This is important because different types of syncope have different restrictions. A summary of the 2007 regulations is outlined in Table 6.1. Readers are advised to check the DVLA website as this information may change.

Special considerations when evaluating syncope in older people

The investigation of syncope is the same in older people as for younger people, with the addition of routine supine and upright carotid sinus massage. A 24-hour ambulatory blood pressure monitor can also be useful to look for post-prandial hypotension or over-treated hypertension.

The evaluation of frail older people who present with recurrent collapses depends on compliance with tests and overall prognosis. Clinical decisions on the value of further evaluation should be made for each individual. Lying and standing blood pressure measurements, carotid sinus message and tilt testing are well tolerated even in frail older people with some cognitive impairment.

The following are common pitfalls when evaluating syncope in older people.

- Collapsing without warning is common with vasovagal syncope or postural hypotension in older people and does not necessarily indicate a cardiac cause. Older people have impaired sympathetic reflexes, which means they do not necessarily experience a typical prodrome of feeling light-headed, hot, nauseated and sweating before collapsing.
- 'Talking nonsense' does not necessarily mean an expressive dysphasia. Brief disorientation while coming round can occur in syncope.
- Syncope while sitting is common in older people, especially after meals. Slumping to one side occurs when muscle tone is lost and does not necessarily indicate a transient ischaemic attack.
- 'I must have tripped' is a common statement made by older people with syncope, who have retrograde amnesia for the event. About one-third of patients who lose consciousness during carotid sinus massage deny they have done so immediately afterwards.

Table 6.1 Driving regulations in the UK for syncope (2007).

Disorder	Group 1 licence (car or motorcycle)	Group 2 licence (bus, lorry) and taxi drivers
Vasovagal and situational syncope	No restrictions	No restrictions
Cough syncope	Driving must cease until liability to attacks has been controlled	Driving must cease and the person must be free of syncope for 5 years
Unexplained syncope* and low risk of re-occurrence (i.e. no abnormality on cardiovascular and neurological examination and normal ECG)	Can drive 4 weeks after the event	Can drive 3 months after the event
Unexplained syncope* and high risk of re-occurrence (i.e. abnormal ECG, structural heart disease, syncope causing injury, occurring at the wheel or whilst sitting or lying, more than one episode in the last 6 months)	Can drive 4 weeks after the event if the cause has been identified and treated. If no cause identified, cannot drive for 6 months	Can drive after 3 months if the cause has been identified and treated. If no cause identified, then licence revoked for 1 year
Loss of consciousness with seizure markers (i.e. strong clinical suspicion of a seizure but no evidence)	Cannot drive for 1 year	Cannot drive for 5 years
Loss of consciousness with no clinical pointers whatsoever (after evaluation by a specialist)	Cannot drive for 6 months	Cannot drive for 1 year

* 'Unexplained syncope' should be the opinion of an experienced doctor. See Figure 6.3 for the evaluation of unexplained syncope.

- Frail older people can appear 'post-ictal' after syncope because they are less able to compensate for brief cerebral hypoperfusion than young people.

Tilt testing

During a tilt test, the patient lies flat for around 10 minutes and is attached to a cardiac and beat-to-beat blood pressure monitor. The patient is then tilted upright at 70° and observed for 30 minutes for symptoms and signs of syncope (see Figure 6.4). If the patient remains asymptomatic, various methods may be used to increase orthostatic stress (e.g. sublingual glyceryl trinitrate or application of lower body negative pressure) and the heart rate and blood pressure response is monitored for a further 20 minutes. The tilt table is also used to perform carotid sinus massage both supine and upright, as one-third of cases of carotid sinus hypersensitivity are missed if the test is only performed supine. Autonomic function tests can also be done in certain patients.

Tilt testing can be useful if the patient's symptoms are reproduced and accompanied by hypotension, bradycardia or both, particularly early in the test (see Figure 6.5). A slow fall in blood pressure after head-up tilt in older people is also commonly observed, and can confirm a suspected diagnosis of postural hypotension despite normal lying and standing blood pressures. More details about tilt testing can be found in the further resources section.

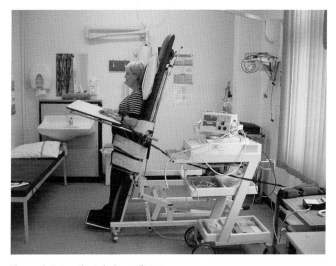

Figure 6.4 A patient during a tilt test.

Use of the implantable loop recorder in older people

The implantable loop recorder (Reveal® device) is an electrocardiogram monitor which is placed subcutaneously under local anaesthesia in a similar way as a pacemaker box. It records the patient's electrocardiogram on a continuous loop and can remain implanted for up to 24 months. It can be activated by the patient after a

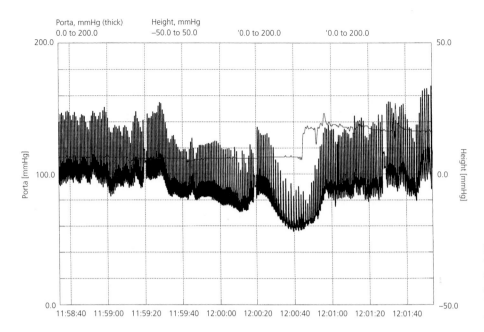

Figure 6.5 Blood pressure readings during a tilt test. This recording shows blood pressure (vertical axis) over time (horizontal axis). Just after time 12:00:20, there is a sudden fall in blood pressure, which recovers quickly as soon as the tilt table is laid flat.

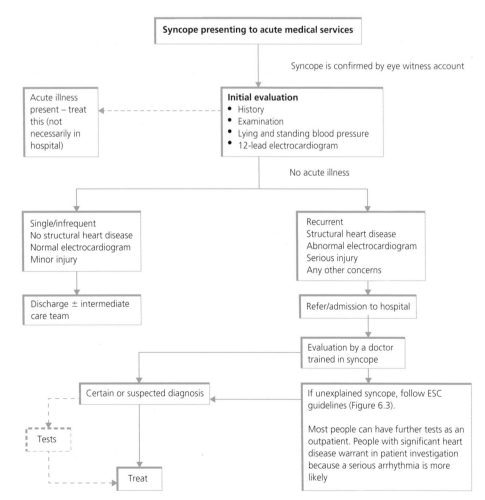

Figure 6.6 When to admit and when to refer patients with syncope. Adapted from: Brignole M, Alboni P, Benditt DG *et al.* The Task Force on Syncope, European Society of Cardiology. *Eur Heart J* 2001; 22(15): 1256–1306.

collapse. The implantable loop recorder has a high diagnostic yield for infrequent events and has a high patient compliance. Indications for an implantable loop recorder include the following.

- Patients with recurrent syncope with structural heart disease in whom arrhythmias are suspected despite negative tests.
- Patients with recurrent unexplained syncope without structural heart disease when understanding the exact mechanism may alter treatment.
- Patients with 'epilepsy' who are not responding to appropriate treatment.

Treatment of recurrent syncope

Figure 6.6 shows when to admit and when to refer patients with syncope. Neurally mediated syncope is treated by patient education and general measures such as ensuring good hydration, avoidance of triggers and exacerbating antihypertensive medication, and increased salt in the diet if the blood pressure is low and there are no other contraindications. Certain patients may benefit from a pacemaker, such as those with cardioinhibitory (bradycardic) carotid sinus hypersensitivity.

Postural (orthostatic) hypotension is treated in a similar way. Very often, reducing or stopping certain medication is all that is required. Box 6.4 shows a list of drugs that commonly cause postural hypotension in older people. Some patients benefit from volume-expanding medication (e.g. fludrocortisone), and severe cases (e.g. in autonomic failure) may require midodrine, a vasoconstrictor drug which can only be prescribed on a named patient basis by a specialist.

The treatment of cardiac arrhythmias and structural cardiopulmonary disease requires referral to a cardiologist.

Box 6.4 **Drugs that commonly cause postural hypotension in older people**

More likely to cause a problem
- Alpha blockers
- Vasodilators (e.g. nitrates)
- Other antihypertensives
- Diuretics
- Psychiatric drugs (e.g. tricyclics, major tranquillisers, benzodiazepines)
- Any drug with anticholinergic properties

Syncope is a common condition and a thorough initial evaluation will often reveal the underlying diagnosis without the need for further tests. It may be the presentation of a serious heart condition, but more commonly, neurally mediated syncope or postural hypotension is the cause.

Further resources

Benditt DG, Blanc J-J, Brignole M, Sutton R, eds. (2006) *The Evaluation and Treatment of Syncope. A Handbook for Clinical Practice*, 2nd edn. [A publication based on the guidelines on management (diagnosis and treatment) of syncope by the European Society of Cardiology.] Blackwell Publishing, Oxford.

Grubb P, Olshansky B, eds. (2005) *Syncope. Mechanisms and Management*, 2nd edn. Blackwell Publishing, Oxford.

The European Society of Cardiology website www.escardio.org

The Driver and Vehicle Licensing Agency website www.dvla.gov.uk

Cooper NA, Feely M. Epilepsy: problems of diagnosis and recommended treatment [prescribing in older people series]. *Prescriber* 2007; 18(5): 72–8. Available from www.escriber.com

CHAPTER 7

Transient Ischaemic Attack and Stroke

Jon Cooper

OVERVIEW

- Transient ischaemic attack (TIA) and stroke are medical emergencies that require urgent assessment
- Patients with a high-risk TIA or stroke should be admitted to hospital
- Stroke unit care significantly reduces death and disability
- Modifying risk factors and starting secondary prevention reduces the risk of subsequent stroke
- Stroke remains a leading cause of death and disability in the UK, so prevention is of the utmost importance

---

Cerebrovascular disease is no longer regarded as an inevitable consequence of old age, but rather a treatable syndrome which is a medical emergency when it presents acutely. Every year in the UK there are about 110 000 patients with new strokes, 30 000 with recurrent strokes and 20 000 with transient ischaemic attacks. This includes 10 000 strokes in adults under retirement age. Overall, 11% of all deaths each year in the UK are attributable to stroke and it is the largest cause of serious adult neurological disability, with about £2.8 billion spent each year on direct care. As the proportion of older people increases, so will the impact of stroke.

The pathophysiology of stroke

Stroke is caused by a sudden disruption to the blood supply to the brain. There are two main types: cerebral infarction and intracerebral haemorrhage, the latter of which includes subarachnoid haemorrhage (see Figure 7.1). Infarction and haemorrhage are not underlying diagnoses, as there are several different mechanisms (see Figure 7.2).

Cerebral infarction results from a blockage of arterial blood supply either by atherothromboembolism to large or small vessels, or embolisation from a proximal source such as the heart, as in atrial fibrillation. Rarer causes such as arterial dissection and inflammatory vasculopathies also occur. Following disruption of cerebral blood flow, there is disturbance to the neuronal electrical activity (reversible) and cellular membrane integrity (irreversible)

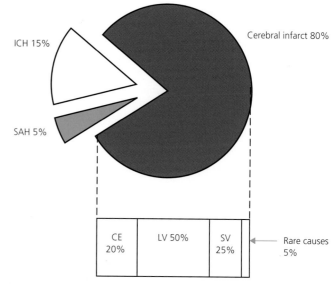

Figure 7.1 Frequency and mechanism of stroke by pathological subtype. ICH, intracerebral haemorrhage; SAH, subarachnoid haemorrhage; CE, cardio-embolic; LV, large vessel; SV, small vessel. From Warlow C *et al. Lancet* 2003; 362: 1212.

through a neurochemical cascade. The 'ischaemic penumbra' is an area of brain that has not passed into the irreversible stage and has the potential to recover. This is the rationale for emergency therapy in cerebral ischaemia. Figure 7.3 shows the computed tomography (CT) appearances of various types of infarct.

Primary intracerebral haemorrhage (ICH) follows a rupture of blood vessels into brain tissue, resulting in direct neuronal injury and cerebral oedema (see Figure 7.4).

Clinical assessment

Stroke and TIA are clinical diagnoses, characterised by the *sudden* onset of a *focal* neurological deficit. It is impossible to reliably differentiate cerebral infarction from cerebral haemorrhage on clinical grounds alone.

The particular symptoms of stroke and TIA depend on which part of the brain is affected and these are listed in Box 7.1. There are also a number of other disorders that may mimic stroke (Box 7.2), but these can often be differentiated by history and physical examination.

The traditional difference between a stroke and TIA is timing. In TIA, neurological symptoms and signs resolve within 24 hours.

ABC of Geriatric Medicine. Edited by N. Cooper, K. Forrest and G. Mulley.
© 2009 Blackwell Publishing, ISBN: 978-1-4051-6942-4.

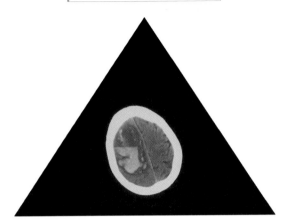

Haemodynamic
Chronic arterial hypertension
Acute arterial hypertension
Drugs e.g. amphetamines, cocaine
Post-carotid endarterectomy

Anatomical
Small vessel disease
Cerebral amyloid angiopathy
Cerebral aneurysm
Arteriovenous malformations
Cerebral venous thrombosis
Mycotic emboli/aneurysms

Coagulopathy
Anticoagulation
Thrombolysis
Antiplatelet drugs
Blood disorders:
    Thrombocytopenia
    Haemophilia
    Leukaemia
    DIC

Figure 7.2 Different mechanisms leading to intracerebral haemorrhage.

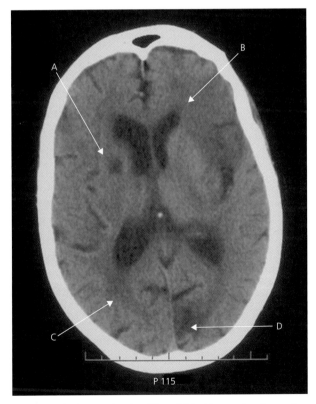

Figure 7.3 CT brain scan showing (A) established lacunar (small vessel) infarct, (B) acute left middle cerebral artery territory infarct, (C) diffuse small vessel disease and (D) established left posterior cerebral artery infarct.

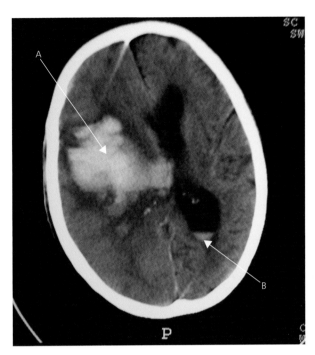

Figure 7.4 CT brain scan showing a large-volume intracerebral haemorrhage (A) in the right cerebral hemisphere, with evidence of intraventricular extension (B).

Box 7.1 **Clinical features of stroke/TIA with arterial territory**

Anterior (carotid) circulation	Posterior (vertebrobasilar) circulation
Cortical dysfunction: dysphasia sensory/visual inattention hemianopia	Cranial nerve palsy Ataxia/incoordination/ disequilibrium* Diplopia* Isolated homonymous hemianopia
Monocular blindness Unilateral weakness Unilateral sensory disturbance	Bilateral visual loss Unilateral/bilateral weakness Unilateral/bilateral sensory disturbance
Dysarthria* Neuromuscular dysphagia*	Dysarthria* Neuromuscular dysphagia*

* Unlikely to be TIA or stroke if symptoms are in isolation.

However, most TIAs last less than 1 hour and those of the eye last for only a few minutes. Many so-called TIAs lasting several hours are actually infarcts (as evidenced on CT scanning).

Our concepts of stroke and TIA are evolving. It is more helpful to think in terms of a 'brain attack', particularly for those assessed within the first few hours of their event, in whom it is unclear whether it will turn out to be a TIA or a stroke. For patients who present with a TIA, it is possible to identify those at the highest risk for stroke using a simple score (see the ABCD2 score in Box 7.3). This is crucial in prioritising patients, organising investigations, modifying risk factors and starting effective secondary prevention (see Box 7.4).

Box 7.2 **Stroke mimics**

- Seizures
- Sepsis with previous stroke (old neurological signs may become more pronounced)
- Cerebral tumour
- Subdural haemorrhage
- Intoxication with alcohol
- Migraine
- Inner ear disease
- Transient global amnesia
- Cervical spondylosis with nerve entrapment
- Functional disorder (rare in old age)

Box 7.3 **The ABCD2 score and subsequent stroke risk**

The National Stroke Strategy suggests that patients with a TIA and score of 5 or more should be admitted to hospital for immediate specialist investigation.

ABCD2	Score	
Age	> 60 years	1
Blood pressure	>140/90 mmHg	1
Clinical features	Unilateral weakness	2
	Speech disturbance alone	1
	Other	0
Duration of symptoms	>60 minutes	2
	10–59 minutes	1
	<10 minutes	0
Diabetes mellitus	Present	1

Risk of stroke after a TIA	ABCD2 score	2-day risk	7-day risk	90-day risk
Low	0–3	1%	1.2%	3.1%
Moderate	4–5	4.1%	5.9%	9.8%
High	6–7	8.1%	11.7%	17.8%

From Johnston SC *et al. Lancet* 2007; 369: 283–92.

Box 7.4 **Risk factors for stroke and TIA**

- Hypertension
- Tobacco smoking
- Diabetes mellitus
- Atrial fibrillation
- Hyperlipidaemia
- Previous stroke or TIA
- Lifestyle and diet
- Peripheral arterial disease
- Ischaemic heart disease
- Male gender
- Advancing age

Box 7.5 **Key questions in suspected TIA or stroke**

1 Is it sudden?
2 Is it focal?
3 Has it resolved?
4 Was there impaired consciousness?

- If the answer to **1–3** is yes, go to ABCD2 score for TIA
- If the answer to **1** and **2** is yes but **3** is no, manage as for stroke
- If the answer to **4** is yes, explore possibility of another diagnosis, e.g. seizure

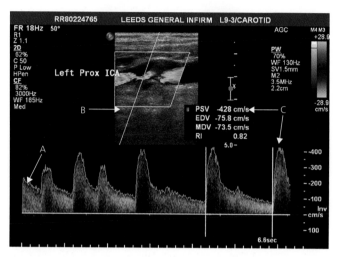

Figure 7.5 Carotid Doppler ultrasound. Carotid Doppler spectrum (A) showing a high-grade stenosis of the left internal carotid. Colour Doppler flow (B) demonstrating mosaic pattern of high flow velocity. The systolic blood flow velocity at the point of maximal narrowing (C) is more than 400 cm/s (normal is less than 100 cm/s).

General management

All patients with a TIA or stroke should be assessed urgently (see Box 7.5). Patients with a TIA and a high ABCD2 score and patients who still have neurological symptoms and signs should be admitted to hospital. Patients with more than one TIA in a week are also considered to be at high risk.

For patients with a high-risk TIA, admission to hospital allows urgent:

- carotid Doppler ultrasound, if the TIA was in the carotid territory (see Box 7.1 and Figure 7.5), and surgery if there is significant stenosis in the symptomatic artery
- risk factor assessment and secondary prevention
- anticoagulation if the patient is in atrial fibrillation
- thrombolysis if the patient has a stroke while in hospital.

Those with lower risk scores or who refuse admission should have their risk factors addressed, be started on antiplatelet therapy and referred to a TIA clinic.

The management of stroke should take place without delay – including neuroimaging, consideration of hyperacute treatment (thrombolysis), initiation of early secondary prevention and admission to organised stroke unit care. This allows medical stabilisation, and monitoring of blood pressure, pulse rate and rhythm,

Box 7.6 **Post-stroke complications**

Neurological	Non-neurological
Progression or stroke completion	Sepsis:
Further stroke	urinary
Haemorrhagic transformation	aspiration pneumonia
Cerebral oedema	Metabolic:
Seizure (partial or generalised)	electrolyte disturbance
Hydrocephalus	hypo-/hyperglycaemia
	dehydration
	Pulmonary embolus
	Cardiac arrhythmia

If a patient becomes more drowsy after a stroke, think of the five Ss: seizures, sepsis, sugar, stroke recurrence and secondary hydrocephalus.

Box 7.7 **Investigations for TIA or stroke**

All patients	Selected patients	Difficult 'syndromes'
FBC	Thyroid function	Vasculitic screen/
Clotting	Troponin	immunology
Urea and electrolytes	Liver function	Echocardiogram
Glucose	Fasting glucose	Transcranial Doppler
Cholesterol	Oral glucose	ultrasound
PV/ESR*	tolerance test	Magnetic resonance
12-lead ECG	Chest X-ray	imaging
CT brain scan	Carotid Doppler	Cerebral angiography
	ultrasound	

* PV, plasma viscosity; ESR, erythrocyte sedimentation rate.

temperature, blood glucose and oxygen saturations (all things which can affect the ischaemic penumbra mentioned earlier). Complications can be identified early (e.g. raised intracranial pressure, aspiration pneumonia – see Box 7.6), specific stroke treatment can be given, and early co-ordinated rehabilitation can begin (see Chapter 11).

There is strong evidence that stroke unit care is more effective than care on general medical wards, reducing death and disability by about 30%.

The management of patients with spontaneous primary intracerebral haemorrhage is generally supportive. Patients on anticoagulants should be considered for treatment with vitamin K or prothrombin complex concentrate, depending on the reason for anticoagulation and the clinical severity of the haemorrhage. There is insufficient evidence to support neurosurgical intervention in most cases, apart from cerebellar haematomas or superficial bleeding in patients who deteriorate neurologically.

Investigations

The investigations for patients with TIA and stroke are shown in Box 7.7.

All patients with a stroke should have CT of the brain. CT accurately differentiates cerebral infarction from haemorrhage (up to 2 weeks) and can identify some conditions that mimic stroke. An immediate scan should be undertaken if:
• thrombolysis is being considered
• subarachnoid haemorrhage is suspected
• there is rapidly deteriorating neurology
• the patient is anticoagulated.
Otherwise CT should be performed as soon as possible within the first 24 hours. *A normal CT scan does not exclude stroke.* Small infarcts may not be seen, and large infarcts may produce only subtle changes on imaging if performed very early.

Thrombolysis in stroke

There is a firm evidence base that cerebral reperfusion with thrombolysis (r-tPA, Alteplase) improves recovery in selected subgroups of stroke patients. Although there is an increase in early mortality from intracerebral haemorrhage, total mortality at 3 months is unchanged, with more patients surviving with less disability. The effect of treatment is time dependent and most benefit is seen when it is given within 3 hours. Patients presenting within this time and in whom rigid inclusion and exclusion criteria are applied can be considered for treatment in stroke centres with specialists trained in thrombolysis.

Secondary prevention

Antiplatelet agents

Antiplatelet agents should be considered the first line of treatment in all patients with TIA and ischaemic stroke, apart from those with a potential cardiac source of embolisation. In terms of *early* secondary prevention, aspirin is the only antiplatelet with proven benefit in acute stroke and though the effect is small, it reduces subsequent death and disability. It should be started as soon as the diagnosis of stroke has been made or within 48 hours if there will be a delay in obtaining CT results. The dose (excluding those with contraindications or who have received thrombolysis) is 300 mg daily by mouth or nasogastric tube, or 600 mg per rectum.

Following the first event, in which a patient is not taking an antiplatelet agent (and in whom there is no high-grade internal carotid artery stenosis for which surgery is being planned), aspirin 300 mg orally once daily should be continued for 2 weeks, reducing to 75 mg once daily *plus* modified-release dipyridamole 200 mg twice daily. This regimen is cost-effective and is superior to aspirin alone in reducing subsequent stroke risk.

When a patient already taking aspirin suffers a 'breakthrough' event, modified-release dipyridamole 200 mg twice daily should be added. Clopidogrel is possibly more effective than aspirin alone in preventing recurrent vascular events, but is not cost-effective as a first-line treatment following TIA or stroke. Patients who are allergic to aspirin or who suffer a 'breakthrough' event on an aspirin–dipyridamole combination should be prescribed clopidogrel 75 mg once daily. There is no current evidence at this time to support the combination of clopidogrel with aspirin or dipyridamole.

Box 7.8 **CHADS2 score for prediction of stroke risk in atrial fibrillation**

C	Congestive heart failure	1
H	Hypertension (systolic >160 mmHg)	1
A	Age >75 years	1
D	Diabetes mellitus	1
S	Previous TIA or stroke	2

Score	Risk classification	Risk per year	Therapy	Dose
0–1	Low	1.9–2.8%	Aspirin	75–300 mg daily
2–4	Moderate	4.0–8.5%	Aspirin or warfarin	INR 2.0–3.0
5–6	High	12.5–18.2%	Warfarin	INR 2.0–3.0

From: Gage *et al. Circulation* 2004; 110: 2287–92.

Anticoagulation

Prophylactic low molecular weight heparin or anticoagulation for atrial fibrillation should not be used in the acute phase of cerebral infarction. Although this treatment leads to a reduction in venous thromboembolism and fewer recurrent ischaemic strokes, there is an increase in symptomatic intracerebral haemorrhage, with no net benefit in reducing recurrent stroke.

The convention is to wait about 14 days after the event before starting anticoagulation. Patients in atrial fibrillation with a recent TIA or cerebral infarct should be considered for long-term anticoagulation with warfarin, particularly if their annual risk of stroke is high (see Box 7.8). This reduces the risk of subsequent stroke by about two-thirds, aiming for a target international normalised ratio (INR) of 2.5 (range 2.0–3.0). Any decision to recommend oral anticoagulation should take into account the risks (major bleeding complications) and benefits (stroke reduction). Oral anticoagulation is not more effective than antiplatelet therapy for patients in sinus rhythm.

Risk factor management

Hypertension is an important modifiable risk factor for stroke. Epidemiological data have shown a linear relationship between arterial blood pressure and stroke. Acute reduction in blood pressure following stroke may cause harm and is subject to ongoing clinical trials. Treatment should begin at least 1 week following stroke, aiming for a blood pressure of less than 140/85 mmHg (130/80 mmHg in people with diabetes).

Cholesterol has a weak but positive association with ischaemic stroke compared to coronary artery disease, but reducing cholesterol to less than 3.5 mmol/L (e.g. with simvastatin 40 mg orally once daily) reduces the risk of stroke and other vascular events by about 25%. There are few data for cholesterol reduction in patients over 82 years of age.

Smoking is an important risk factor and all patients who smoke should be advised to stop. Dietary advice is also important and includes salt restriction, five portions of fresh fruit and vegetables a day, oily fish once a week, low saturated fat diet, and moderate alcohol consumption, as well as increased physical exercise and weight reduction if necessary.

Carotid revascularisation

There is good evidence that carotid endarterectomy reduces stroke risk in patients with a recent carotid territory TIA or non-disabling stroke, if they are fit and willing for surgery. The benefit of surgery is greater if done early and when there is a higher degree of stenosis. If the event occurred within 2 weeks, surgery is of benefit with a greater than 50% stenosis, but after this time the benefit is only seen in a 70–99% stenosis and the absolute risk reduction for stroke declines rapidly. Those with carotid *occlusion* require no vascular intervention.

Outcome following stroke

Death and disability remain an unfortunate consequence of stroke with a mortality of 12% at 7 days, 19% at 30 days and 31% at 12 months. Impaired consciousness, cerebral haemorrhage, location and size of the lesion, age and medical co-morbidities all affect mortality. Poor functional outcome is associated with cognitive decline, poor motivation, urinary incontinence, severe motor weakness, and perceptual, proprioceptive and postural problems. Around one-third of stroke survivors will suffer a recurrence.

Further resources

Hankey GJ. (2002) *Stroke: your Questions Answered*. Churchill Livingstone, London.

Brown MM, Markus H, Oppenheimer S. (2006) *Stroke Medicine*. Taylor and Francis Group, London.

Royal College of Physicians. (2004) *National Clinical Guidelines for Stroke*, 2nd edn. Prepared by the Intercollegiate Stroke Working Party. RCP, London. www.rcplondon.ac.uk/pubs/books/stroke/index.htm

Scottish Intercollegiate Guidelines Network. (2002; updated 2005) Management of patients with stroke: rehabilitation, prevention, and management of complications and discharge planning. www.sign.ac.uk/guidelines/published/index.html#CHD

Johnston SC, Rothwell PM, Nguyen-Huynh MN *et al*. Validation and refinement of scores to predict very early stroke risk after transient ischaemic attack. *Lancet* 2007; 369: 283–92.

Acknowledgements

The author would like to thank Dr Tony Goddard and Dr David Kessle (consultants in neuroradiology and vascular radiology respectively) for their help with image selection and Edward Taylor (vascular radiographer). Dr Richard Fuller kindly reviewed the manuscript.

CHAPTER 8

Dementia

John Wattis & Stephen Curran

OVERVIEW

- Dementia is common in old age, especially extreme old age
- People with dementia should be assessed thoroughly
- The general management of people with dementia in health and social care should be improved
- All aspects of the patient's physical health and surroundings need to be taken into account to provide the best care

Introduction

The risk of developing dementia rises with increasing age (see Table 8.1). An ageing population means that dementia is on the increase. This should allow planners and politicians to forecast needs and hopefully to develop services. In the UK there are currently over 750 000 people with dementia. This is projected to rise to over 850 000 by 2010 and 1.8 million by 2050. Because of its economic impact, dementia is an important target for diagnostic and therapeutic research and development. To the clinician it presents a challenge in accurate differential diagnosis and management, and is also a factor in managing other illnesses in older people.

Definitions

Dementia is defined as an acquired, global and progressive impairment of mental function. Being *acquired* distinguishes it from learning disability, being *global* distinguishes it from focal disorders such as stroke or Parkinson's disease (though both of these can result in dementia) and being *progressive* distinguishes it from non-progressive impairment, for example following trauma, or reversible impairment in delirium.

Dementia can also be defined as a syndrome due to disease of the brain, usually of a chronic or progressive nature in which there is, in the absence of clouding of consciousness, disturbance of multiple higher cognitive functions (Box 8.1).

Table 8.1 Prevalence of dementia by age. From Jorm AF, Korten AE, Henderson AS. The prevalence of dementia: a quantitative integration of the literature. *Acta Psychiatrica Scandinavica* 1987; 76: 465–79.

Age (years)	Prevalence (%)
<65	Rare
65–69	1.4
70–74	2.8
75–79	5.6
80–84	11.1
>85	23.6

Box 8.1 **Higher cognitive functions disturbed in dementia**

- Memory
- Thinking
- Orientation
- Comprehension
- Calculation
- Learning capacity
- Language
- Judgement

Types of dementia

Dementia is a *syndrome* with a variety of causes (Table 8.2). Of these causes, Alzheimer's disease is the most common, followed by various types of vascular dementia (which have the same risk factors as stroke – see Chapter 7) and dementia with Lewy bodies (DLB). The metabolic 'dementias', although rare, are important because of their potential reversibility (e.g. hypothyroidism). Other causes of dementia are also rare and usually manifest at a younger age. There are some rare genetic variants of Alzheimer's disease with early onset and increased familial risk. Early-onset Alzheimer's is also a feature of Down's syndrome.

Symptoms and differential diagnosis

Deficiencies in memory, orientation, judgement, comprehension and learning (especially in new situations) are the most common

---

ABC of Geriatric Medicine. Edited by N. Cooper, K. Forrest and G. Mulley.
© 2009 Blackwell Publishing, ISBN: 978-1-4051-6942-4.

Table 8.2 Different types of dementia.

Type of dementia	Approximate % of cases
Alzheimer's disease	55% (includes a considerable number of mixed Alzheimer–vascular cases)
Vascular dementia (subtypes: acute onset, multi-infarct, subcortical)	20%
Dementia with Lewy bodies (DLB)	15%
Frontotemporal dementia syndromes (e.g. Pick's disease)	5%
Other dementias (e.g. metabolic 'dementias' like vitamin B12 and thyroid deficiency, Creutzfeldt–Jakob disease, Huntington's disease, Parkinson's disease, AIDS-related dementia)	5% (though small in number, these are important to diagnose because some may be reversible, some are inherited and others are potentially transmissible)

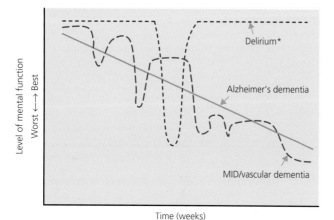

Figure 8.1 Time courses of delirium vs dementia. MID, multi-infarct dementia.

*In delirium, some patients may be left with new cognitive impairment even after recovery, and others will have underlying dementia.

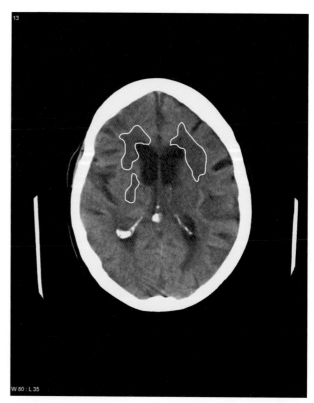

Figure 8.2 Typical CT appearances in vascular dementia. The image shows an area of low attenuation (darker) within the posterior limb of the right internal capsule (bottom left circle) which is an old infarct. There are also two further areas of low attenuation around both frontal horns of the lateral ventricles (top two circles). This is due to small vessel ischaemic damage, often termed 'periventricular white matter changes', due to diffuse cerebrovascular disease. The ventricles and sulci are also prominent, indicating some atrophy which may be normal for the patient's age.

presenting symptoms of dementia. The term 'confusion' is often used by relatives or doctors but is imprecise and should be clarified, or avoided. Cognitive testing will often reveal deficiencies in these and other areas. The Mini Mental State Examination (MMSE) accesses a variety of these areas (orientation, registration, attention, calculation, recall and language) and gives a rough indication of severity (see further resources section). However, poor intelligence and education, or acute illness causing delirium, are factors that can affect the result.

The time course of the illness is important in differential diagnosis. Figure 8.1 shows the typical time courses of delirium (discussed further in Chapter 3), Alzheimer's disease and multi-infarct dementia, the most common form of vascular dementia. DLB shows an overall gradual decline similar to Alzheimer's but with much greater fluctuation in performance during the day. Extrapyramidal signs, susceptibility to the extrapyramidal side-effects of antipsychotics and prominent visual hallucinations are also characteristic of DLB. Subdural haematoma may also give a fluctuating picture, but often with more obvious transient impairment of conscious level.

The course of multi-infarct dementia is described as stepwise with periods of sudden decline interspersed with periods of relative stability. Findings of hypertension, atrial fibrillation, diabetes, or neurological signs and symptoms suggestive of cerebrovascular disease support the diagnosis. Computed tomography (CT) of the brain (Figure 8.2) may confirm the presence of vascular lesions, but does not exclude the possibility of mixed vascular and Alzheimer's dementia.

Investigations

The metabolic 'dementias' may be excluded by appropriate laboratory tests (see Box 8.2). Blood tests for syphilis, serum lipids and HIV should be considered in high-risk populations. A CT scan of the brain should be routine in early-onset dementia and should be requested urgently in the presence of:

- a rapid unexplained deterioration
- neurological signs or symptoms
- a recent head injury
- urinary incontinence or gait apraxia (in which the feet seem to stick to the floor) early in the illness, suggesting normal-pressure hydrocephalus which may be treatable
- an atypical presentation of dementia.

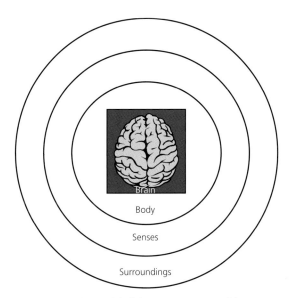

Figure 8.3 An interactive model of dementia. For successful treatment, all these interacting aspects of a person's function should be considered.

Management

Assessment in practice

The assessment and management of dementia is a multidisciplinary exercise. A useful framework is given in Figure 8.3. To ensure the best possible outcome for someone with dementia, function should be optimised in each area.

When the onset of cognitive impairment is sudden or when there is sudden worsening of existing confusion, there is likely to be a medical cause such as infection, metabolic disturbance, stroke or medication (e.g. drugs with anticholinergic properties or sedatives). Thorough physical examination and urgent investigations are indicated, followed by appropriate treatment. Once this has been dealt with, a re-assessment should determine the cause and extent of any remaining cognitive impairment, associated sensory impairment and relevant social and family factors.

When cognitive impairment presents more gradually, there is time to make a comprehensive assessment from the start. Increasingly this is a function of specialist memory services associated with mental health services for older people and follows Royal College and National Institute for Health and Clinical Excellence (NICE) guidelines (see further resources section).

Person-centred care

The general management of dementia should follow a person-centred approach – this recognises that some of the handicaps we see in people with dementia are caused or made worse by their environment. Admission to hospitals poses particular problems, as acute hospital care focuses on the medical rather than the psycho-social needs of demented people.

People with dementia benefit from being with family or friends, and in familiar surroundings whenever possible. If they have to be admitted to hospital or intermediate care, someone they know and trust should accompany them to explain (repeatedly, if necessary) what is going on. Lack of comprehension is made worse when allowances are not made for the difficulties people with dementia have about learning, remembering and adapting to change. These aspects are considered in more detail in the NICE guidelines and in books such as *Dementia Reconsidered* (see further resources section). The medical role may focus on diagnosis, review of medication, management of physical health problems and appropriate prescribing, but it is essential for the doctor to ensure that other areas are considered and that appropriate services are delivered to improve function and reduce carer strain.

Dementia requires long-term care planning as well as acute management. Older people with dementia are vulnerable to abuse and doctors must know how to deal with suspected abuse.

Pharmacological management

Pharmacological management in dementia consists of:
- specific anti-dementia drugs
- medication for co-existing physical problems
- medication for behavioural disorders.

The cholinesterase inhibitors donepezil, rivastigmine and galantamine opened a new era in the treatment of Alzheimer's dementia. However, a recent NICE guideline has stated that the benefits are only sufficient to justify treatment of moderate Alzheimer's. Thus patients with mild dementia have to wait until they deteriorate before they can have treatment and patients with severe dementia are likely to have treatment withdrawn (though most local services reinstate treatment if there is marked deterioration on withdrawal).

The treatment of vascular dementia is the same as that for the secondary prevention of stroke (see Chapter 7).

Patients with dementia may not complain about physical illness in a way that is easy to understand. Their health should therefore be kept under regular review. They may not be good at remembering to take medication. Prescribers should simplify the medication regimen as far as possible, seek to explain to patients and carers the purpose and importance of any prescribed medication and co-operate with carers to optimise compliance.

Person-centred care minimises the risk of behaviour disturbance. Behavioural problems in dementia may be due to:
- an acute illness causing delirium
- chronic problems (e.g. constipation or pain)
- undiagnosed or untreated depression
- sensory deprivation (e.g. flat hearing aid battery, inadequate spectacles)

- carer strain
- inadequately trained or over-busy staff.

A simple behavioural analysis using 'ABC' (antecedents, behaviour, consequences) may be useful. Understanding the causes is more likely to lead to appropriate remedial action, rather than the prescription of antipsychotic or sedative medication. When antipsychotics are indicated they should be initiated by specialists and given in the lowest effective dose for the shortest possible time.

Social, emotional and spiritual support

Social, environmental and spiritual support can be offered to patients with dementia and their carers in the following ways.

- Their involvement in decisions about their care.
- Information about their disease and what they can do to help themselves.
- Information about financial benefits (see Chapter 15).
- Practical support with day-to-day living.
- Respite care.
- Support in maintaining social life and religious practice.
- Emotional support in coping with the effects of the disease.
- If necessary, long-term care.

People with dementia are not well served by present health or social services. We can all play our part in changing this for the better.

Further resources

The Alzheimer's Society. For people with dementia, their relatives and carers and professionals. www.alzheimers.org.uk

Curran S, Wattis J, eds. (2004) *Practical Management of Dementia: a Multi-Disciplinary Approach.* Radcliffe Publishing, Oxford.

Folstein MF, Folstein SE, McHugh PR. 'Mini mental state': a practical method for grading the cognitive state of patients for the clinician. *J Psyc Res* 1975; 12(3): 189–98.

Kitwood T. (1997) *Dementia Reconsidered: The Person Comes First.* Open University Press, Buckingham.

National Institute for Health and Clinical Excellence. (2006) Dementia: supporting people with dementia and their carers in health and social care. Clinical Guideline 42. NICE, London. www.nice.org.uk

Royal College of Psychiatrists Council Report CR119. (2005) *Forgetful but not forgotten: assessment and aspects of treatment of people with dementia by a specialist old age psychiatry service.* RCPsych, London.

CHAPTER 9

Urinary Incontinence

Eileen Burns & Anne Siddle

OVERVIEW

- Incontinence is common among older people
- The impact of incontinence is significant
- Incontinence is not an inevitable consequence of ageing
- It can be treated after a proper assessment
- A lot can be done to promote the comfort and dignity of older people with intractable incontinence

---

Urinary incontinence is a common condition that affects people of all ages and both sexes. Changes occur in the urinary tract with ageing (see Box 9.1) that predispose to incontinence in older people.

Incontinence is defined as 'any involuntary leakage of urine'. Although more common, incontinence is *not* inevitable in old age, and much can be done to prevent and treat it. A positive attitude and a thorough assessment can mean maintaining dignity and independence for most people.

The prevalence and impact of incontinence

Up to 1 in 5 women and around 1 in 10 men over the age of 65 suffer from incontinence. The prevalence increases with increasing age and co-morbidity. Two-thirds of care home residents are incontinent of urine. However, with variations in definitions and under-reporting due to embarrassment, the prevalence of incontinence is probably an underestimate.

Incontinence can significantly affect a person's wellbeing. People with incontinence restrict their social activities. Carer strain is common and incontinence is second only to dementia as an initiating factor in admission to a care home. Soiled clothing, bed linen and soft furnishings have to be laundered and replaced frequently, resulting in an increased financial burden. Incontinence overall costs the NHS over £420 million per year (approximately 1% of the total NHS budget).

ABC of Geriatric Medicine. Edited by N. Cooper, K. Forrest and G. Mulley.
© 2009 Blackwell Publishing, ISBN: 978-1-4051-6942-4.

Box 9.1 Changes in the urinary tract with ageing

- Shortening of the urethra
- Post-menopausal atrophy of the urothelium
- Reduced bladder sensation
- Reduced detrusor muscle function
- Increased residual bladder volume
- Less effective urethral closure

Box 9.2 Drugs that can worsen or precipitate incontinence

- Diuretics
- Sedatives
- Alpha blockers
- Any drug with cholinergic properties

Co-morbidities and incontinence

Diseases that are prevalent in older age can affect continence. Any disability affecting vision, mobility, dexterity or cognition may have an adverse effect on continence, especially if an individual has a problem with urgency of micturition.

Treatments for diseases may also have the unintended effect of precipitating incontinence. Some examples are given in Box 9.2. Patients with dementia may have incontinence because of either the disease process itself or its treatment, for example with cholinergic drugs, which can worsen an overactive bladder.

Patients with poorly controlled diabetes may have polyuria. Less commonly, patients with hypercalcaemia, hypokalaemia or diseases of the pituitary gland may present with urinary frequency or incontinence. There is also an association between incontinence and falls.

Assessment

There are different types of urinary incontinence and symptoms vary in nature and severity (see Table 9.1). Each type is treated differently, so it is important to assess which type of incontinence a person has. This is based on the history and examination – urodynamics (specialised tests) are rarely needed.

Table 9.1 Types of urinary incontinence in older people.

Type of incontinence	Definition	Causes	Symptoms
Urge	The complaint of involuntary leakage of urine accompanied or immediately preceded by urgency	Overactive bladder (OAB)	Frequency, urgency, nocturia. Unable to delay voiding
Stress	Involuntary leakage of urine on effort or exertion, coughing or sneezing	Weak pelvic floor muscles, incompetent urethra. Raised intra-abdominal pressure	Leaks urine on exertion, coughing, laughing, sneezing
Mixed	The complaint of involuntary leakage associated with urgency and also with effort or exertion	OAB and weak pelvic floor	Combination of the above
Voiding problems	The generic term for obstruction during voiding, characterised by increased detrusor pressure and a reduced urinary flow rate	Prostatic hypertrophy, detrusor failure (neurogenic bladder), faecal impaction	Hesitancy, poor stream, post-micturition dribble. May have large residual urine volume. Impaired bladder sensation
Functional incontinence	Inability to toilet independently	Extrinsic factors such as immobility, confusion, inability to access toilet facilities, medications etc.	Incontinent if carer unavailable or unable to communicate needs, or cannot get to toilet

Box 9.3 **Key components of a continence assessment**

- History of onset and duration of problems
- Symptom sorter (see Box 9.4)
- Previous medical, surgical and obstetric history
- Medications
- Assessment of functional abilities
- Examination of the abdomen, rectum (and perineum/vagina in women)
- Urinalysis
- Urea and electrolytes, glucose, calcium (and prostate-specific antigen in men)

In addition, patients are asked to keep a 'bladder diary'. It is also very important to ask about bowel problems, as constipation leading to faecal loading can cause urinary problems.

In a continence clinic, further assessments are typically undertaken, which include:
- post-micturition bladder scan (to look for evidence of voiding problems)
- measurement of urine flow (using a special commode)
- quality of life score
- measurement of body mass index.

There are five main types of urinary incontinence in older people:
- urge incontinence (or over-active/unstable bladder)
- stress incontinence
- mixed incontinence (both urge and stress)
- voiding problems (due to obstruction or a neurogenic bladder)
- functional incontinence (due to an inability to get to the toilet, or confusion).

All older people presenting with urinary incontinence should be offered an assessment. Box 9.3 shows the key components of this. Any member of the healthcare team can initiate it and there are useful diagnostic tools available to facilitate this.

As well as the assessment outlined in Box 9.3, a simple 'symptom sorter' is useful in determining the type of incontinence (Box 9.4). A bladder diary, detailing volumes of urine voided, wet episodes, type and amount of fluids taken is also useful – for example, caffeine and citrus drinks can exacerbate bladder instability. A physiotherapist or occupational therapist can help if patients have mobility problems or difficulty accessing toilet facilities in their own home.

A physical examination of the abdomen for palpable masses or urinary retention, and the rectum for faecal impaction, is important. In males, a rectal examination should include an assessment of the prostate. In females, an examination of the perineum and vagina is useful to identify a prolapse or atrophic vaginitis (a reddened excoriated vulva) and to assess for weak pelvic floor muscle contraction – all of these problems contribute to incontinence and can be treated.

Urinalysis can detect infection or diabetes. In continence clinics, a portable bladder ultrasound scanner is used to assess whether patients have a significant post-micturition volume of urine that may indicate voiding problems (see Figure 9.1). Figure 9.2 shows a portable urine flow meter.

Treatment

General measures
General measures that can help promote continence in older people include:
- staying active
- losing weight if necessary
- drinking water rather than caffeine or alcohol.

Box 9.4 **Symptom sorter**

Yes to the following suggests STRESS INCONTINENCE
- I leak when I cough, laugh, sneeze, exercise
- I leak small amounts of urine
- I know when I have leaked
- Only my pants get wet
- I leak during sex

Yes to the following suggests URGE INCONTINENCE
- I have an urgent need to pass urine
- I sometimes do not reach the toilet in time
- I get up more than twice at night
- I pass urine more than 7 times a day
- I get very wet

Yes to the following suggests VOIDING PROBLEMS
- My urine flow stops and starts
- Sometimes I cannot pass urine straight away
- I sometimes feel I have not emptied my bladder properly
- I have a feeling of fullness in my bladder area
- I get frequent urine infections

Yes to the following suggests FUNCTIONAL INCONTINENCE
- I have lots of health problems
- I have problems with memory and concentration
- I need help to move about
- I have problems adjusting my clothing
- I have a feeling of sadness, depression, loneliness

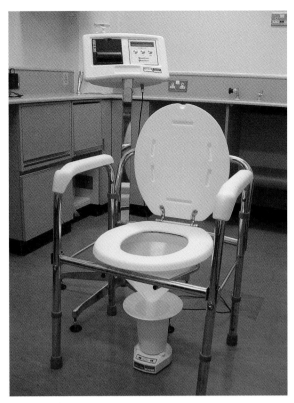

Figure 9.2 Portable urine flow meter used in a continence clinic.

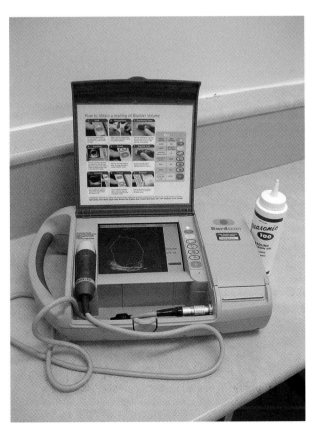

Figure 9.1 A portable bladder scanner.

In hospitals or care homes, toilets should be clearly identified and walking aids or assistance available if needed. If an older person has an impaired memory, carers should prompt them regularly to use the toilet. Carers of people with dementia should be aware of non-verbal cues such as agitation or wandering, which may mean the person needs the toilet.

Urge incontinence (or over-active/unstable bladder)

With urge incontinence, patients cannot wait. They have to pass urine as soon as they feel an urge to go. They may also complain of frequency and nocturia. 'Bladder drill' (going to the toilet at regular intervals) followed by 'bladder training' (gradually extending the length of time between these intervals) is of benefit for patients with this condition.

Drug treatment may be required and there are a number of anti-cholinergic treatments that act on the detrusor muscle of the bladder. Many drugs are non-selective anticholinergic agents, but newer drugs have been developed that specifically target the muscarinic receptors found predominantly in the bladder, with a lower incidence of side-effects, an important consideration in older people.

The National Institute for Health and Clinical Excellence (NICE) guidance in 2006 recommended the use of immediate-release oxybutynin, but this is not well tolerated in older people as it is a non-specific anticholinergic agent. Anticholinergic side-effects include:
- confusion
- dry mouth
- blurred vision

- constipation
- urinary retention
- postural hypotension
- oesophageal reflux.

Extended-release preparations, or antimuscarinic drugs such as tolteradine, are often more acceptable, with a lower incidence of side-effects. These preparations also have the advantage of once-daily dosage. Trospium chloride (a newer antimuscarinic drug) is useful in patients with cognitive impairment, as it has fewer cognitive side-effects.

If treatment for an over-active/unstable bladder is unsuccessful, patients may be offered botulinum toxin which is injected into the detrusor via cystoscopy. This procedure has to be repeated and there is a lack of research on its efficacy. Surgery to augment the bladder is rarely performed nowadays.

Stress incontinence

With stress incontinence, patients leak urine whenever they cough, sneeze, laugh or even stand up. This is usually because of weak pelvic floor muscles in women, as a result of childbirth. The mainstay of treatment for this condition is pelvic floor muscle exercises, which can produce improvement in symptoms even in relatively frail older patients. The patients must be clear about the muscle groups they are trying to strengthen and they must be committed to a programme of regular exercise to obtain and maintain improvement. Working with a trained physiotherapist is the best way to achieve this. Patients with very low pelvic floor tone may benefit from augmentation of their exercise programme with either vaginal cones (Figure 9.3) or biofeedback (in which vaginal cones are connected to a computer that senses muscle contraction and helps the patient contract the right muscles correctly).

If exercise treatment fails then duloxetine may be tried. This is a selective serotonin and noradrenaline re-uptake inhibitor which has some efficacy in patients with stress incontinence, although it is not always tolerated in older patients.

Surgery is also an option for stress incontinence. Even quite frail patients may be able to undergo a TVT (tension-free vaginal tape) or TOT (trans-obdurator tape) procedure. However, outcome data specific to older people suggest that voiding problems, tape divisions and urinary tract infection are more common postoperatively than in younger patients. Periurethral bulking procedures that involve injection of collagen or gels are less invasive but may need to be repeated.

Mixed incontinence

Urge and stress incontinence may co-exist. Usually, it is easy to tell this on the basis of a history and bladder diary. Initial treatment on the basis of a clinical assessment is reasonable, but if the diagnosis is unclear or the patient fails to respond to first-line treatment, urodynamic tests (Box 9.5) may be useful.

Voiding problems

Voiding problems occur in both sexes and are caused by:
- outflow obstruction e.g. enlarged prostate, urethral stricture, constipation
- neurogenic bladder e.g. diabetes, neurological diseases.

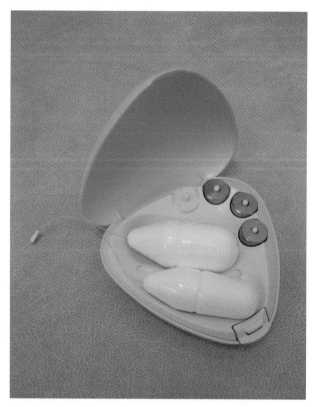

Figure 9.3 Vaginal cones. Vaginal cones are a set of increasing weights which the patient practises holding inside her vagina. This strengthens the pelvic floor muscles.

Box 9.5 **Urodynamics**

Urodynamics is a series of tests performed in a laboratory.
- Filling cystometry: the bladder is filled with saline via a catheter and a volume–pressure graph is produced (a cystometrogram, CMG). This measures bladder compliance and stability.
- Flow/pressure studies: these are usually performed straight after CMG. The patient is asked to urinate and detrusor pressure is measured at maximum flow.
- Videocystourethography: the above tests combined with X-ray screening, used in complex cases.

Patients with voiding problems present with hesitancy and a poor stream. However, chronic outflow obstruction also affects the detrusor muscle and causes bladder instability, so in a man who presents with urge incontinence, anticholinergic treatment may worsen matters if the underlying problem is an enlarged prostate causing outflow obstruction – the underlying cause should be looked for and treated.

Voiding problems are treated with drugs to improve bladder emptying, surgery to remove an obstruction, or urinary catheterisation (intermittent or long term).

Drugs to improve bladder emptying include alpha blockers for prostatic hypertrophy which act on the bladder sphincter, but cause postural hypotension which can be a problem. Anti-testosterone tablets (e.g. finasteride) are an alternative, but these take at least

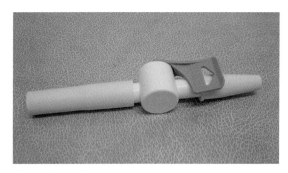

Figure 9.4 Catheter valve.

3 months before an effect is noticed. These drugs are often given together.

If catheterisation is required the preferred option is intermittent self-catheterisation. This is associated with a lower risk of infection and is usually more acceptable to patients. Long-term catheterisation may be the only usable method for some patients, *but is a last resort as a treatment for incontinence.* A valve should be used if possible, rather than a drainage bag (see Figure 9.4) in order to maintain normal bladder filling and reduce infection risk. If a bag is to be used then leg bags are preferable.

When treatment does not work

If treatment for incontinence is unsuccessful there is a huge range of aids and appliances to help the older person cope with their symptoms and remain active and independent. Most of these are available on prescription. A continence nurse specialist can assess the patient and help to decide which aids and appliances would be most effective. This is important, because incorrect appliances or the wrong type of pad may be ineffective and reinforce the myth that incontinence is a problem that cannot be managed.

Further resources

Department of Health. (2000) *Good Practice in Continence Services.* DH, London. www.dh.gov.uk

Department of Health. (2001) *National Service Framework for Older People.* DH, London.

Royal College of Physicians of London. (2006) *National Audit of Continence Care for Older People.* RCPL, London. www.rcplondon.ac.uk

National Institute for Health and Clinical Excellence. (2006) Guidelines for the management of urinary incontinence in women. *Clinical Guideline 40.* NICE, London. www.nice.org.uk

CHAPTER 10

Peri-operative Problems

Kirsty Forrest

OVERVIEW

- Older people with acute surgical problems tend to present atypically
- They have an increased incidence of peri-operative complications
- Particular geriatric problems include under-nutrition, pressure sores, post-operative cognitive dysfunction and a decline in mobility and function
- There is evidence that outcomes for older people are improved when they are proactively cared for by a multispecialty team

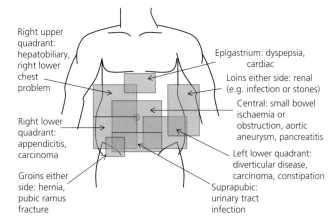

Figure 10.1 An approach to the older patient with acute abdominal pain – site of the pain. Remember that older people may have pain which is less severe than would be expected, and the site of pain may be less well localised and more diffuse than in a younger person.

Assessing older patients who may require surgery can be challenging. They are more likely to present with atypical symptoms and signs. The risks vs benefits of any surgical procedure have to be weighed carefully, and peri-operative care is more likely to be complicated and prolonged. Yet there is good evidence that outcomes can be improved when older people receive tailored care before, during and after surgery.

Atypical presentation

The following considerations, outlined in Chapter 1, are important when assessing older surgical patients.
There is often:
- Multiple pathology
- Atypical presentations
- Reduced physiological reserve
- Impaired immunity
- Difficulty weighing the benefits vs risks of treatment
- Capacity or communication problems.

When older people present with an acute illness, they may have more than one acute diagnosis (e.g. intra-abdominal pathology and fast atrial fibrillation), as well as more than one chronic problem, diagnosed or otherwise.

Older people represent a high percentage of patients with acute abdominal pain. They often present late, have a disproportionately severe pathology compared with the pain they complain of, and their physical findings are less sensitive and less specific. Morbidity and mortality among older patients with abdominal pain is higher than in other age groups.

Because of reduced physiological reserve and impaired immunity, symptoms and signs that one would expect to find in a younger person may be absent (e.g. tachycardia, fever, raised white cells and abdominal rigidity). Evaluating an older patient with acute abdominal pain can be difficult and an experienced surgeon should be involved *early* in the process.

Figures 10.1 and 10.2 describe an approach to the older patient with acute abdominal pain.

Peri-operative complications

Older people have an increased incidence of peri-operative complications, especially after emergency surgery. This is because of age-related physiological differences and reduced physiological reserve that affect all body systems (see Table 10.1). Some peri-operative problems may go unrecognised because of their atypical presentation.

The care of the elderly surgical patient was highlighted in a National Confidential Enquiry into Peri-operative Death

ABC of Geriatric Medicine. Edited by N. Cooper, K. Forrest and G. Mulley.
© 2009 Blackwell Publishing, ISBN: 978-1-4051-6942-4.

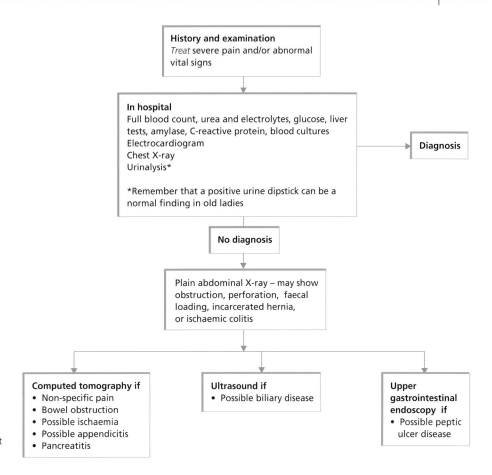

Figure 10.2 An approach to the older patient with acute abdominal pain – general strategy.

Table 10.1 Effects of ageing on physiological reserve.

	Physiological effects	Diseases that are more prevalent
Cardiovascular system	↓Cardiac output and stroke volume ↑Systemic vascular resistance ↓Ability to raise heart rate Cardiac conduction defects	Coronary artery disease Hypertension Heart failure Valvular heart disease
Respiratory system	↓Functional residual capacity V/Q mismatch ↓Response to hypoxia and hypercapnia	Chronic obstructive pulmonary disease
Nervous system	↓Cerebral blood flow ↓Peripheral nerve function	Peripheral neuropathy Autonomic neuropathy Stroke Dementia Parkinson's disease
Renal	↓Renal blood flow and glomerular filtration rate ↓Renal clearance of drugs	Chronic renal disease
Metabolic	↓Body metabolism ↓Response to hypothermia	Diabetes Thyroid disease
Hepatic	↓Hepatic blood flow ↓Hepatic excretion of drugs	

(NCEPOD) report in 1999, which looked at over 1000 patients over the age of 90. The recommendations of the report are shown in Box 10.1.

The NCEPOD report highlighted the following areas.

Fluid management

The mismanagement of fluid prescribing was a contributory factor in many cases of post-operative morbidity and mortality. Patients were given either too little or too much fluid,

Box 10.1 **NCEPOD report 'Extremes of Age' 1999**

Recommendations
- Fluid management in elderly patients is often poor; it should be accorded the same status as drug prescribing. Multidisciplinary reviews to develop good local working practices are required.
- A team of senior surgeons, anaesthetists and physicians needs to be closely involved in the care of elderly patients who have poor physical status and high operative risk.
- The experience of the surgeon and anaesthetist need to be matched to the physical status of the elderly patient, as well as to the technical demands of the procedure.
- If a decision is made to operate on an elderly patient then that must include a decision to provide appropriate post-operative care, which may include high dependency or intensive care support.
- There should be sufficient, fully staffed, daytime theatre and recovery facilities to ensure that no elderly patient requiring an urgent operation waits for more than 24 hours once fit for surgery. This includes weekends.
- Elderly patients need their pain management to be provided by those with appropriate specialised experience in order that they receive safe and effective pain relief.
- Surgeons need to be more aware that in older people, clinically unsuspected gastrointestinal complications are commonly found at post mortem to be the cause, or contribute to the cause, of death following surgery.

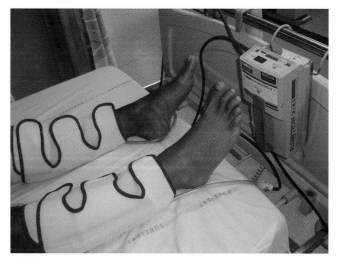

Figure 10.3 Thromboembolism prophylaxis. This patient is wearing an intermittent compression device, which provides mechanical thromboprophylaxis.

Box 10.2 **Factors associated with the development of pressure ulcers**

- Long wait before surgery
- Intensive care unit stay
- Longer surgical procedure
- General anaesthesia

The above factors were from studies in fractured neck of femur patients. Larger studies in general hospital inpatients also found the following significant factors.
- Increasing age
- Low body mass index
- Low serum albumin
- Female gender
- Poor functional status

with inadequate assessment and monitoring – vital in this age group.

Nutrition

Early nutrition after surgery is associated with reduced mortality and length of stay in hospital. The report recommended that feeding should be started as early as possible after surgery.

DVT prophylaxis

Older patients have an increased risk of death from thromboembolism following emergency admission to hospital. Many studies have shown a reduced incidence of deep vein thrombosis (DVT) and pulmonary embolism if prophylaxis is given (see Figure 10.3).

Pain control

The report highlighted the inaccurate perception that older people do not feel as much pain, which may be due to an inability to express it, or patients not wanting to bother staff. Judicious use of opioid analgesics is often required and works well.

Oxygen therapy

Oxygen therapy for 3–4 days after major surgery, especially at night, reduces the incidence of post-operative cardiac complications (e.g. myocardial infarction).

Particular geriatric problems associated with surgery

Under-nutrition

Improving peri-operative nutrition improves outcome in certain surgical patients (e.g. those with fractured neck of femur). However,

under-nutrition is common among older people admitted to hospital, so they start at a disadvantage. Malnourished people stay in hospital for longer, are three times more likely to develop peri-operative complications, and have a higher mortality. Two-thirds of older people are at risk of *becoming* malnourished while in hospital. The UK Department of Health report *Improving Nutritional Care* (see further resources section) was largely in response to successful campaigning by charities for older people.

Pressure ulcers

Pressure ulcers occur when patients are immobile or in bed for prolonged periods of time. The presence of pressure ulcers is associated with prolonged hospital stay and delayed rehabilitation, and may lead to sepsis. Box 10.2 lists the factors associated with the development of pressure ulcers.

Pressure ulcers can usually be prevented. Identification of at-risk patients, skilled nursing care, adequate pain control, hydration and nutrition, the use of pressure redistribution devices, and correct positioning are all important aspects of care.

Box 10.3 **Risk factors for:**

Early POCD	Prolonged POCD
Increasing age	Increasing age
Duration of anaesthesia	
Post-operative infections	
Respiratory complications	

Box 10.4 **Peri-operative complications and death in the over 80s**

Type of operation	Post-operative complications (%)	Mortality (%)
Elective	25	4.6
Emergency	68	31

Post-operative cognitive dysfunction

Post-operative cognitive dysfunction (POCD) is the term used for delirium following anaesthesia with no other apparent cause, for example infection or medication. It is a transient, usually short-lived disorder of memory, cognition and attention. When other causes of delirium have been excluded, a diagnosis of POCD can be made. It is thought to be related to the interaction of anaesthetic agents and the neurotransmitters involved with cognition. The prognosis is good in most patients. However, in some it can be prolonged or lead to complications (see Chapter 3).

Initially, POCD was believed to be a side-effect of cardiac bypass surgery, but an international study found an incidence of 26% at 1 week and 10% at 3 months in older patients undergoing non-cardiac surgery. Box 10.3 lists the risk factors for the development of POCD.

These findings have partly led to the increased use of regional anaesthesia for surgery whenever possible in older people. However, some patients develop POCD after regional anaesthesia, suggesting that other factors are involved.

Decline in ability to perform activities of daily living

Many patients suffer a decline in mobility and ability to perform activities of daily living (ADLs) after admission to hospital for an acute illness. Studies have found that the following premorbid factors are independently associated with decline in ability to perform ADLs:

- cognitive impairment
- depression
- malnutrition
- unsteadiness
- older age.

Peri-operative care programmes that incorporate the principles of comprehensive geriatric assessment (see chapter 1) reduce disability and need for admission to a care home.

Pre-optimisation

Major surgery, especially emergency surgery, places a huge physiological stress on the body. Older people, and those with cardiorespiratory disease, may not have the ability to increase their cardiac output sufficiently to meet increased demands, and this group of patients faces the greatest risk of peri-operative complications and death (Box 10.4). 'Pre-optimisation' refers to physiological measurements and treatment before surgery, specifically aimed at improving a person's cardiac output and oxygen delivery. Pre-optimisation improves patient outcome, especially in high-risk surgical patients.

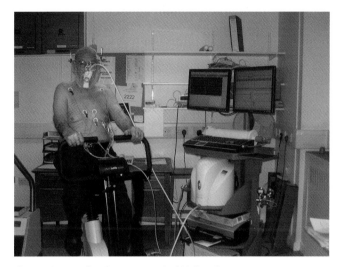

Figure 10.4 Cardiopulmonary exercise (CPX) testing.

At a basic level, pre-optimisation involves measuring a patient's vital signs, performing key blood tests (e.g. haemoglobin and electrolytes), and aiming to restore these as far towards normal as possible before surgery. This is so the patient can mount his or her best compensatory response during the peri-operative period. Simple interventions include oxygen therapy and fluid resuscitation. For elective surgery, a physician may be involved in optimising a chronic disease before admission.

At a more sophisticated level, pre-optimisation involves admission to a high dependency unit (HDU) or intensive care unit (ICU) where cardiac output and oxygen delivery can be measured and manipulated by fluid resuscitation and drugs.

For elective surgery, risk prediction scores can predict overall peri-operative morbidity and mortality, but these do not provide individualised information that can help to plan care for an individual patient. Cardiopulmonary exercise (CPX) testing is increasingly being used to provide an objective measure of a person's physiological reserve (Figure 10.4). Studies have focused on those over the age of 60, or with a history of heart disease. The patient is asked to pedal on an exercise bicycle while measurements are taken that calculate the anaerobic threshold (AT). The test does not require high physical stress or motivation on the part of the patient and accurately predicts those who are at higher risk of peri-operative cardiovascular complications. This information can be used to triage patients to ICU, HDU or ward care, if the patient and surgeon decide to go ahead.

Box 10.5 **Factors in deciding on admission to ICU**

The decision to admit an elderly patient to ICU should be based on:
- co-morbidities
- nature and severity of the acute illness
- pre-hospital functional status, especially mobility and social independence
- patient preferences.

Intensive care for older people

As a group, patients over the age of 80 have poorer outcomes following admission to ICU, compared with younger people. ICU mortality in the over 80s is 27% overall in the UK, and about 50% of patients over the age of 70 will die within 3 months of discharge. However, prognosis depends more on the severity of the acute illness and the patient's previous functional ability, rather than age itself. Severe sepsis and brain injury have particularly poor outcomes.

There is little evidence on which to predict long-term outcomes for physical and cognitive function after discharge from ICU. Studies show that at least one-third of survivors are more disabled in their ability to perform activities of daily living. For selected patients, the evidence is that ICU and HDU care is worthwhile. However, many doctors do not know the preferences of their patients regarding invasive ventilation or cardiopulmonary resuscitation. Information from outcome studies may help doctors and patients make better informed decisions.

The factors that should be taken into account when deciding on admission to ICU are listed in Box 10.5.

The effectiveness of multispecialty teams

Several studies have shown reduced hospital stay and morbidity following elective surgery in older people by using a multispecialty care approach. They have used various methods affecting all or part of the pre-, peri- and post-operative care period (see Table 10.2).

A multispecialty team approach for surgery in older people combines the following:
- pre-operative patient education
- pre-optimisation
- fast-track surgery
- attenuation of surgical stress
- optimised pain relief
- early mobilisation
- nutritional support.

Delivering these requires a co-ordinated approach between geriatricians, surgeons and anaesthetists, as well as other disciplines (e.g. physiotherapy) and hospital managers.

Harari *et al.* in a cohort study (see further resources section) showed improvements in pressure ulcers, pain control, mobilisation and reduced length of stay in elderly patients undergoing elective orthopaedic surgery. They used a multispecialty team targeting

Table 10.2 Care pathway for the surgical elderly patient: interventions and the multidisciplinary team.

When	What	Who
Pre-operatively	Assessment Patient education Medical optimisation Nutrition	General practitioner Nurse Surgeon Anaesthetist Geriatrician Physiotherapist
Peri-operatively	Type of anaesthetic Fluids and monitoring ICU or high dependency unit Minimally invasive surgery	Nurse Surgeon Anaesthetist Geriatrician Physiotherapist
Post-operatively	Pain relief and fluids Nutrition Post-operative complications Early mobilisation Rehabilitation	Nurse Surgeon Anaesthetist Geriatrician Occupational therapist Physiotherapist

most of the above aspects of care. However, they did not look at surgical or anaesthetic techniques, which also affect outcome for older people.

In the UK, a new speciality of orthogeriatrics has evolved to improve care for elderly trauma patients. Different models exist, all of which involve a geriatrician sharing the care of patients with fractures, predominantly fractured neck of femur. This involves pre-optimisation, post-operative care, rehabilitation and discharge planning in a multidisciplinary team. Other important aspects of care include reducing subsequent falls risk and investigations and treatment for osteoporosis.

All successful models of care for older surgical patients adopt an integrated approach, involving the surgical team and a geriatric multidisciplinary team. Experience worldwide has shown that an unintegrated approach results in poorer overall outcomes.

Further resources

Cooper N, Forrest K, Cramp P. (2006) Optimising patients before surgery. In: *Essential Guide to Acute Care*, 2nd edn. Blackwell Publishing, Oxford.

National Confidential Enquiry into Perioperative Death. (1999) *Extremes of Age.* NCEPOD, London. www.ncepod.org.uk/pdf/1999/99full.pdf search 'extremes of age'

Department of Health. (2007) *Improving Nutritional Care. A Joint Action Plan from the Department of Health and Nutrition Summit Stakeholders.* DH, London. www.dh.gov.uk/publications

National Institute for Health and Clinical Excellence. (2005) The management of pressure ulcers in primary and secondary care. *Clinical Guideline* CG29. NICE, London. www.nice.org.uk

Harari D, Hopper A, Dhesi J, Babic-Illman G, Lockwood L, Martin F. Proactive care of older people undergoing surgery (POPS): designing, embedding, evaluating and funding a comprehensive geriatric assessment service for older elective surgical patients. *Age Ageing* 2007; 36(2): 190–6.

CHAPTER 11

Rehabilitation

Lauren Ralston & John Young

OVERVIEW

- Illness in older people often has functional consequences
- Randomised controlled trials show that rehabilitation is effective in improving function and independence
- Rehabilitation is a multidisciplinary process, with specific treatment goals
- Barriers to successful rehabilitation include unidentified medical problems that can be treated

Introduction

Illness in older people often has functional consequences, especially in relation to mobility and self-care. This was recognised by one of the pioneers of geriatric medicine – Marjory Warren (Figure 11.1). She took over the care of several hundred chronically sick, bedridden, 'incurables' in the West Middlesex Hospital in the 1930s and devised a novel programme that was patient-centred and involved multidisciplinary team working. So successful was her approach that most of these incurable patients improved sufficiently to be discharged from hospital. This was the beginning of the specialty of geriatric medicine and her novel approach would today be recognised as rehabilitation.

What is rehabilitation?

Rehabilitation is a complex intervention that aims to address the functional, psychological and social consequences of ill-health in a context that values and promotes independence. It requires a multidisciplinary team, identifies specific individualised treatment goals, and measures progress against these goals.

The World Health Organization (WHO) International Classification of Functioning, Disability and Heath (ICF) describes the consequences of illness and provides an important framework within which the rehabilitation process can be understood (Box 11.1). The WHO ICF framework requires a medical diagnosis

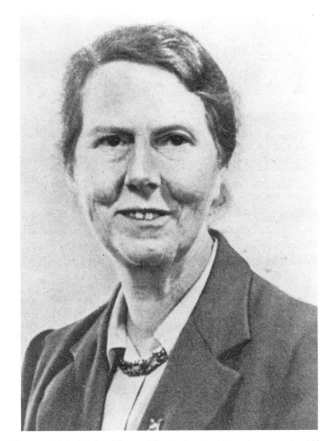

Figure 11.1 Dr Marjory Warren. 'The treatment of long-stay cases should be undertaken by a team whose central theme is optimism and hope. It is wise to get elderly folk up as soon as their physical condition warrants, and it is of great value to their morale to get them dressed in their own clothing as soon as possible.' From Marjory Warren. Care of the chronic sick. *Lancet* 8 June 1946. Picture reproduced with the permission of the British Geriatrics Society.

Box 11.1 **WHO International Classification of Function (1991)**

- Body functions: the physiological functions of body systems (including psychological functions)
- Impairments: problems in body function or structure such as a significant deviation or loss
- Activity: the execution of a task or action by an individual
- Participation: involvement in a life situation

ABC of Geriatric Medicine. Edited by N. Cooper, K. Forrest and G. Mulley.
© 2009 Blackwell Publishing, ISBN: 978-1-4051-6942-4.

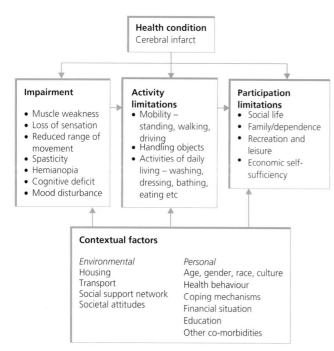

Figure 11.2 WHO International Classification of Function (ICF) using the example of a person with a cerebral infarct affecting a parietal lobe.

(the impairments), while examining the functional consequences (activity limitations, formerly known as disability), and set in the context of the person's daily life (participation limitations, formerly known as handicap). There is often discordance between impairments, activity limitations and participation limitations because of mediating environmental and personal factors. Figure 11.2 provides an example for a person who has a cerebral infarct affecting a parietal lobe.

Who is rehabilitation for?

Activity limitation, or disability, is strongly related to increasing age. This reflects the increasing prevalence of common disabling conditions: stroke, arthritis, heart failure, chronic lung disease, fractured hip and peripheral vascular disease. There are around 1.3 million disabled older people in England and Wales. This is 16% of those aged over 65 years. Nearly all disabled older people, even those categorised as severely disabled, live in their own homes, but many rely on formal and informal support. Rehabilitation can improve the quality of life for these people and make them less dependent on other people. There is randomised controlled trial evidence that rehabilitation interventions can improve outcomes for older people with the following conditions:

- falls
- arthritis of the knees
- Parkinson's disease
- stroke
- chronic lung disease
- old age and multiple conditions (frailty)
- long-term care home residents.

Who provides rehabilitation?

Rehabilitation is provided by a multidisciplinary team (MDT). Core members of this team include the following.

Nurses and support staff – enable patients to be as independent as possible, even though this is usually more time-consuming than completing tasks for them. This is facilitated by ensuring that patients are dressed and are wearing appropriate footwear, and that hearing aids, dentures and glasses are worn if needed.

Doctors – have a lead role in establishing an accurate diagnosis of the underlying and associated conditions, and in optimising their medical management.

Physiotherapists – are skilled at assessing and managing problems of muscles, movement and mobility. Key aims of physiotherapy are to improve balance, flexibility, strength and stamina, often by practising everyday activities such as walking, transferring and climbing stairs.

Occupational therapists – optimise daily living activities and may recommend the use of different aids to assist rehabilitation or maintain independence.

Speech and language therapists – assess and treat speech (e.g. dysphasia, dysarthria) and swallowing impairments.

Social workers – provide access to benefit and allowance advice, and can co-ordinate home support services.

Other staff may need to be involved, depending on the specific needs of the individual patient (Figure 11.3).

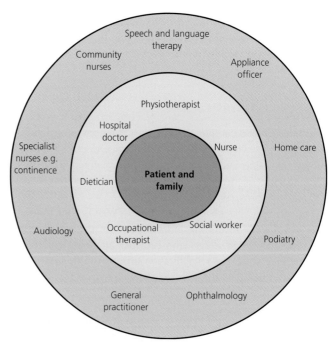

Figure 11.3 Members of the multidisciplinary team.

Box 11.2 **The rehabilitation process**

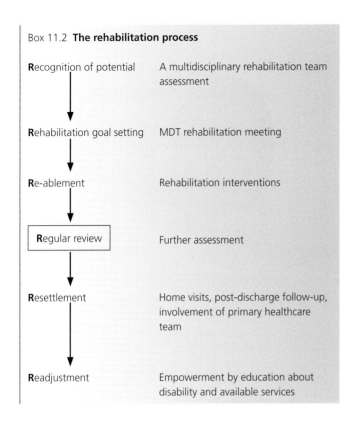

Recognition of potential	A multidisciplinary rehabilitation team assessment
Rehabilitation goal setting	MDT rehabilitation meeting
Re-ablement	Rehabilitation interventions
Regular review	Further assessment
Resettlement	Home visits, post-discharge follow-up, involvement of primary healthcare team
Readjustment	Empowerment by education about disability and available services

How is rehabilitation organised?

Effective rehabilitation requires several steps (Box 11.2) and requires some key functions described below. Omission of any of these key functions will jeopardise the success of the rehabilitation process.

Assessment – by each member of the MDT to identify the diseases and their consequences, best expressed in terms of impairments, activity limitations and participation limitations.

Co-ordination – each member of the MDT will have a different perspective of the issues. These need to be shared and formulated into an action plan. This is usually achieved through a regular MDT meeting.

Leadership – at the MDT meeting, someone needs to assume the role of a team leader to co-ordinate information, achieve a consensus on rehabilitation priorities and goals and agree tasks.

Communication – an important aspect of the MDT meeting is to ensure that decisions are documented and are discussed fully with the patient and close supporters.

Rehabilitation goals – arise from the assessment process as discrete steps within the overall aims of the rehabilitation plan. They can be short or medium term and are most effective when there is significant patient and carer involvement. Rehabilitation goals should be SMART, that is:

> *Specific*: who will do what, when and how often.
> *Measurable*: so that it is clear when the goal has been achieved.
> *Achievable*: but challenging enough to stretch the patient.
> *Relevant*: to what the patient wishes to achieve.
> *Time limited*: to maintain focus on patient improvement.

Standardised rehabilitation measures

Many standardised rehabilitation measures have been developed. Ideally, measures should be valid (i.e. measure what they are supposed to measure), reliable (give the same result for the same patient when repeated), and sensitive to clinical change – but there is no perfect rehabilitation measure. A commonly used generic measure is the Barthel Index (Box 11.3), which measures independence across 10 daily living activities with a score range of 0 (dependent) to 20 (independent). It is rather insensitive to clinical changes and has a low ceiling – patients may score the maximum of 20 points but still have activity limitations in areas not covered by the index, such as cooking or trips outside.

Box 11.3 **The Barthel Index**

Assesses the level of dependence for 10 activities of daily living. The maximum score is 20. The higher the score, the more independent the person is.

Feeding	2 = independent 1 = needs help 0 = unable
Bathing	1 = independent 0 = dependent
Grooming	1 = face/hair/teeth all alone 0 = dependent
Dressing	2 = independent 1 = needs help but can do at least half 0 = dependent
Bowels	2 = continent 1 = occasional accidents, needs help with enemas 0 = incontinent
Bladder	2 = continent, manages own catheter 1 = occasional accidents, needs help with catheter 0 = incontinent
Toilet	2 = independent 1 = needs help 0 = dependent
Transfers from bed to chair	3 = totally independent 2 = minimal help needed 1 = able to sit with major help 0 = needs to be lifted/hoisted
Walking	3 = independent for 50 metres with or without an aid 2 = needs help of a person 1 = independent with a wheelchair 0 = immobile
Stairs	2 = independent 1 = needs help 0 = unable

Adapted from Mahoney FI, Barthel D. Functional evaluation: the Barthel Index. *Maryland State Medical Journal* 1965; 14: 56–61.

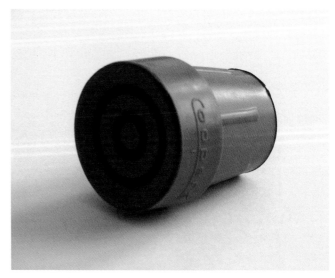

Figure 11.5 A walking stick ferrule (rubber tip).

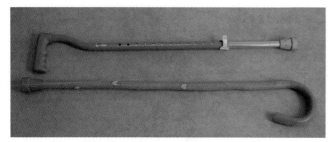

Figure 11.4 Crook and straight-handle walking sticks.

Gait assessment

Limitation of mobility is a common consequence of many chronic
conditions affecting older people and adversely affects quality of
life. Understanding gait assessment is therefore a useful clinical
skill. Much can be learnt from careful observation of balance and
gait using the standardised approaches listed in Box 11.4 (see also
Chapter 4).

Walking sticks

Walking sticks transmit a proportion of body weight through the
upper rather than the lower limb, thus reducing forces through an
unstable or painful joint. This can improve balance, reduce postural sway and increase confidence. Walking sticks are commonly
single ended but may have three (tripod) or four (quadripod)
feet to improve stability. The choice of handle can improve performance: a straight handle with finger grips is preferable as it
improves grip and reduces pressure on the hand; however, a 'crook'
is often preferred by patients as it allows the user to hook it over the
arm when not in use (Figure 11.4). The stick should ideally be used
on the contralateral, unaffected side if the aim is to reduce sway
(e.g. in a hemiparesis), or to reduce weight through a painful joint
(e.g. osteoarthritis of the hip). The length of the stick should be the
distance from the wrist crease to the floor when the arm is resting
at the side of the body. The ferrule or rubber tip (see Figure 11.5)
should be checked regularly for wear.

Walking frames

Walking frames promote an upright posture, provide stability and
reduce the weight transmitted through painful legs. Two main types
exist: the Zimmer frame (four legs, no wheels) and rollator frames
with wheels. The Zimmer frame with its four rubber tips provides
superior stability but this is at the cost of an abnormal, stop/start
gait pattern that tends to force the user to lean backwards when
lifting the frame forwards. In contrast, rollator frames promote a
smoother, striding, more natural gait pattern as demonstrated by
a doubling of gait speed compared to the Zimmer. Studies show
that increased gait speed is correlated with improved balance, fewer
falls and less fear of falling. Additionally, the energy cost of using a
wheeled frame is half that of a Zimmer frame.

A delta frame, or tri-wheeler, is another type of wheeled frame. It
has a single front wheel which swivels and two unidirectional back
wheels. It promotes greater stride length and speed, and is often
preferred by users because of its superior manoeuvrability. Finally,
the gutter frame is a large, cumbersome frame that allows the user
to lean heavily forward by resting their forearms in horizontal gut-
ters and offers maximum stability when the legs are very weak
and/or painful (Figure 11.6).

Daily living aids

Many daily living aids are available. Careful assessment to define the
key patient and carer problems is needed before the most appropriate aid can be selected. Instruction and training following selection
has been shown to improve their effectiveness. Examples of items
commonly required are wheelchairs, special seating, kitchen and
bathing aids, chairs and orthoses (insoles, shoe modifications, support collars, lumbar supports and splints). Such devices promote
independence for the patient but may also help protect the patient
and carer from injury (Figure 11.7).

Type of frame	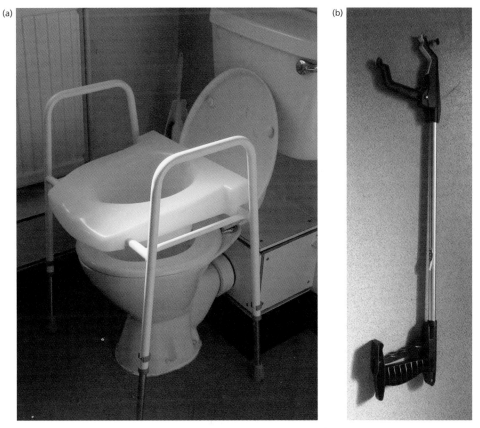Zimmer frame	Rollator	Delta frame	Gutter frame
Advantages	Rubber tips and wide base give increased stability Aid of choice to reduce weight bearing	Normal or striding gait pattern Aid of choice for people with a tendency to lean backwards and in Parkinson's disease	Striding gait pattern Highly manoeuvrable Brakes Greater stride length and speed versus two-wheeled rollator	Increased stability Grip not essential
Disadvantages	Abnormal, stop/start gait pattern	Small wheels unsuitable for use on carpets Requires good weight-bearing ability	Less stable than frames Brakes dependent on wrist strength	Large cumbersome frame
Example of use	Osteoarthritis of the knee or hip	Stroke, post-fall syndrome and Parkinson's disease	Parkinson's disease	Severe pain and weakness in legs

Figure 11.6 Types of walking frame. 'Zimmer' is the name of a manufacturer, but the four legs, no wheels walking frame is commonly referred to by this name.

(a)

(b)

Figure 11.7 (a) Toilet aid and (b) grabber (which helps patients to reach for objects).

Box 11.5 **The Geriatric Depression Scale (GDS 15)**

Used as a screening tool to identify depressive symptoms in the elderly. Consists of 15 Yes/No questions; 1 mark is given for each answer in **bold** below.

1 Are you basically satisfied with life? Y/**N**
2 Have you dropped many of your activities and interests? **Y**/N
3 Do you feel that your life is empty? **Y**/N
4 Do you often get bored? **Y**/N
5 Are you in good spirits most of the time? Y/**N**
6 Are you afraid something bad is going to happen to you? **Y**/N
7 Do you feel happy most of the time? Y/**N**
8 Do you often feel helpless? **Y**/N
9 Do you prefer to stay at home rather than going out and trying new things? **Y**/N
10 Do you feel you have more problems with your memory than most? **Y**/N
11 Do you think it is wonderful to be alive now? Y/**N**
12 Do you feel pretty worthless the way you are now? **Y**/N
13 Do you feel full of energy? Y/**N**
14 Do you feel that your situation is hopeless? **Y**/N
15 Do you think that most people are better off than you are? **Y**/N

Score   0–4   no depression
          5–10   mild depression
          11+   severe depression

Advantages: quick test, takes 5–10 minutes, well tolerated, sensitivity 80%.
Disadvantages: moderate specificity of 60%.
A four-point scale consisting of questions 1, 3, 6 and 7 is also in use. A score of 1 or more suggests depression.

From Yesavage JA, Brink TL, Rose TL *et al.* Development and validation of a geriatric depression screening scale: a preliminary report. *J Psychiatric Res* 1983; 17: 37–49.

Barriers to rehabilitation

Some patients may not progress as expected. Common reasons include the following.

Unidentified medical problems such as anaemia, heart failure, under-treated pain and adverse effects of medication.

Unidentified depression – mood disorders are commonly associated with physical disease in older people. The geriatric depression scale (GDS) can be used for screening purposes (Box 11.5).

Unidentified dementia – impaired memory and concentration may impede rehabilitation techniques that rely on learning and carry-over. Screening for cognitive impairment is advisable using a standardised assessment measure (e.g. the Mini Mental State Examination – see Chapter 8).

Time – patients can only recover at a rate that is appropriate to their physical and psychological condition and some patients will require a longer period of contact with rehabilitation services.

Where should rehabilitation take place?

The location of rehabilitation services varies between geographical areas. There is considerable randomised trial evidence to support the following:
- hospital-based rehabilitation within elderly care services
- stroke unit rehabilitation
- community falls services
- community stroke services.

There is also a trend towards improved outcomes from trial evidence for:
- day hospitals
- community hospitals
- some hospital-at-home services in which patients receive home support and therapy in their own homes.

There are concerns over inferior outcomes associated with care home-based rehabilitation and nurse-led units.

Rehabilitation is one of the success stories of geriatric medicine. Acute and chronic medical conditions in older people commonly lead to reduced function and activities of daily living. With a proper assessment, older people with the potential to improve can be identified and effectively treated.

Further resources

Lee SD, George J. (2007) Gait disorders in the elderly. In: Rai GS, Mulley GP, eds. *Elderly Medicine: a Training Guide*, 2nd edn. Churchill Livingstone, London.

Elmamoun M, Mulley G. Walking sticks and frames for patients with neurological disorders. *Pract Neurol* 2007; 7: 24–31.

Mulley G, ed. (1991) *More Everyday Aids and Appliances*. BMJ Books, London.

Gutenbrunner C, Ward AB, Chamberlain MA, eds. (2007) White book on physical and rehabilitation medicine in Europe. *Journal of Rehabilitation Medicine* 39: 1–48. Can be found at the International Society of Physical and Rehabilitation Medicine website. www.isprm.org/publications/Whitebook.pdf

CHAPTER 12

Palliative Care

Lucy Nicholson & Suzanne Kite

OVERVIEW

- Palliative care is the holistic care of patients with advanced disease and a limited prognosis
- Palliative care is not just for patients with cancer
- All doctors provide palliative care, but specialist palliative care services are available for patients who need it
- Symptom control is an important aspect of palliative care
- End of life decisions should be discussed in advance whenever possible

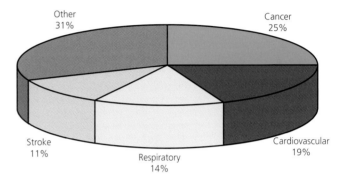

Figure 12.1 Causes of death in the UK.

Around 1% of the UK population dies each year but only 25% of these die from cancer. Figure 12.1 shows the other common causes of death, which include heart failure, chronic respiratory diseases and stroke. Although most people say that they would prefer to die at home, over half will die in hospital. Most people who die are older, which is why palliative care is an important aspect of geriatric medicine.

Definitions

The World Health Organization (WHO) defined palliative care in 2005 as 'the approach that improves the quality of life of patients and their families facing the problems associated with life-threatening illness, through the prevention and relief of suffering by means of early identification and thorough assessment and treatment of pain and other problems – physical, psychosocial and spiritual.'

Palliative care:

- provides relief from pain and other distressing symptoms
- affirms life and regards dying as a normal process
- intends neither to hasten nor postpone death
- integrates the psychological and spiritual aspects of patient care
- offers a support system to help patients live as actively as possible until death
- offers a support system to help the family cope during the patient's illness and their own bereavement

- uses a team approach to address the needs of patients and their families
- enhances quality of life, and may also positively influence the course of the illness
- is applicable early in the course of an illness, in conjunction with other therapies that are intended to prolong life, e.g. chemo- or radiotherapy, and includes investigations needed to better understand and manage distressing clinical complications.

Palliative care requires a multidisciplinary team. Good communication skills are needed to allow patients to tell their own story, discover their preferences for involvement in decision-making and goals of care, and to impart bad news sensitively and honestly (Figure 12.2). Attention to detail is vital, especially with symptom management.

Who provides palliative care?

Most patients receive palliative care from their general practitioners and/or hospital teams. End of life initiatives, such as the Gold Standards Framework and Liverpool Care Pathway for the Dying, have been implemented to support palliative care in these settings (Box 12.1). Referral to specialist palliative care teams should be considered for patients with physical, psychological, social or spiritual needs that cannot be met by their current healthcare teams.

Specialist palliative care (SPC) services are needs based rather than diagnosis based. They include hospices, as well as community and hospital palliative care teams. Hospices provide inpatient services

ABC of Geriatric Medicine. Edited by N. Cooper, K. Forrest and G. Mulley.
© 2009 Blackwell Publishing, ISBN: 978-1-4051-6942-4.

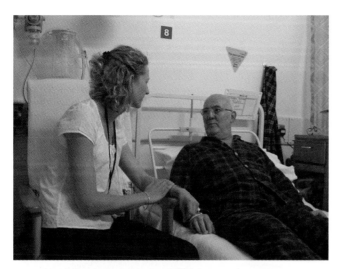

Figure 12.2 Effective communication skills are needed.

Box 12.1 The Gold Standards Framework and Liverpool Care Pathway for the Dying

Gold Standard Framework
- Local community-based system to improve and optimise organisation and quality of care for patients in the last year of life
- Inclusion criteria are all patients who are expected to die in the next year
- Focuses around communication, co-ordination, control of symptoms, continuity (including out of hours), continued learning, carer support and care in the dying phase
- Advance care planning, symptom relief and home support become priorities and targets for quality improvement
- Further information is available at www.goldstandardsframework. nhs.uk

Liverpool Care Pathway
- Transfers best practice for care of the dying in a hospice environment to other care settings
- Inclusion criteria are dying patients with advanced progressive disease with no reversible cause
- Multiprofessional team must agree the patient is dying
- Includes proactive prescribing for common end of life symptoms – pain, nausea and vomiting, excessive respiratory secretions and agitation
- Addresses spiritual care and carers' needs
- Further information available at www.lcp-mariecurie.org.uk

Box 12.2 Special considerations in palliative care for older people

The patient
- Impaired homeostasis (see Chapter 1)
- Cognitive impairment is common
- Symptoms such as pain and insomnia may be seen as 'normal' consequences of ageing
- Activities of daily living are affected more by the same symptom burden than in younger patients

The family
- Older carers, who may not be in good health
- Many patients live alone

The disease
- Increased co-morbidities
- Prognostication is more difficult in non-cancer diagnoses such as chronic obstructive pulmonary disease and end-stage heart failure

Drugs
- Increased number of drugs – therefore higher potential for interactions
- Different pharmacokinetics and pharmacodynamics (see Chapter 2)
- Renal impairment is common
- Concordance may be a problem

Communication
- Hearing loss and visual impairment are common
- Subjective assessment of symptoms requires intact cognition
- Preferred decision-making styles vary with age

Palliative care in older people

The majority of patients requiring palliative care are old, and special consideration needs to be given to their assessment and management because of differences in physiology, co-morbidities and social circumstances. Box 12.2 outlines some of the differences that need to be taken into account.

Symptom management

Symptoms are common at the end of life. Approximately 70% of cancer patients and 65% of patients with non-malignant diseases will experience pain during the course of their illness. Pain and other symptoms should be considered as a total experience, with physical, psychological, social and spiritual components. The pharmacological management of pain uses the stepwise approach of the WHO pain relief ladder, starting with non-opioid analgesics and progressing to increasingly strong opioids, ensuring that drugs are prescribed both regularly *and* as required (see Figure 12.3).

Morphine remains the opioid analgesic of choice for moderate to severe cancer pain, but interindividual variability in absorption, metabolism and excretion may lead to a poor analgesic response or signs of toxicity in up to one-third of patients. In this situation a switch to a different kind of opioid will be necessary.

Neuropathic pain is only partially opioid responsive and usually requires the addition of co-analgesics such as amitriptyline or gabapentin. Nerve blocks can also be considered in difficult pain.

for patients requiring management of complex needs, terminal care or rehabilitation, with an average length of stay of approximately 2 weeks. Many patients are discharged home following a hospice stay. Day care, bereavement support and complementary therapies may also be available.

Community and hospital SPC teams have a mainly advisory role. They also have an important role in education. SPC services have expertise in the management of complex symptoms, whether physical and/or psychological, including pain that is difficult to manage, prescribing at the end of life, and can also offer an outside perspective or second opinion.

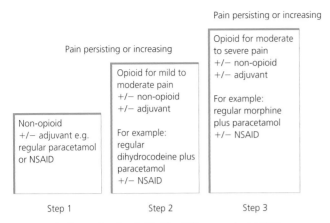

Figure 12.3 The WHO pain relief ladder. PRN, as required; NSAID, non-steroidal anti-inflammatory drug.
Non-steroidals should usually be prescribed with a proton pump inhibitor in older people.

In palliative care:

1 Prompt oral administration of drugs for pain should be initiated in the order shown, until the patient is free of pain.

2 Other drugs (adjuvants) may be needed for neuropathic or bone pain, and for anxiety and poor sleep which can also affect pain.

3 Drugs should always be taken regularly rather than PRN.

This simple 'three-step approach' is 80–90% effective. Specific surgical treatments or radiotherapy may also be indicated. From www.who.int/cancer/palliative/painladder/en

Up to two-thirds of cancer patients will experience nausea and vomiting. The choice of anti-emetic is determined by the cause of the symptoms. Excellent and concise summaries of the management of nausea and vomiting are available in introductory palliative care texts (see further resources section), and local guidelines may also be available, e.g. through Regional Cancer Networks. Anti-emetics sometimes need to be started parenterally, via a continuous subcutaneous infusion, until symptoms are controlled and the patient is able to absorb the drug orally.

Breathlessness and other symptoms should be asked about directly. Patients often do not volunteer information about anorexia, fatigue, insomnia and mouth problems, thinking they are an inevitable consequence of their illness. However, acknowledgement and explanation can help and where treatments are available they can have a significant impact on quality of life.

Box 12.3 shows some of the questions to ask of a patient in a palliative care situation, Box 12.4 gives some tips on symptom management in palliative care, and Figure 12.4 shows how palliative care symptoms can be the result of several factors, and therefore their management involves consideration of the total picture. More information on treatment for difficult symptoms can be found in the further resources section.

Estimating prognosis

Estimating prognosis is vital in palliative care. It helps to determine appropriate treatment options. Patients and families need to make plans about future care and prepare for death. Access to various services and benefits are dependent upon a person's prognosis. In the UK, patients are entitled to receive the higher rate of disability

Box 12.3 Questions to ask of a patient in a palliative care situation

Questions about	Possible courses of action
Pain (remember there may be more than one type of pain, so consider each one in turn)	See the WHO pain relief ladder. Certain pains such as neuropathic pain, liver capsule pain, constipation pain, or headaches due to raised intracranial pressure require specific treatments
Bowels	Many painkillers cause constipation, which must be treated
Nausea and vomiting	Treat with appropriate anti-emetics. Specific causes (e.g. bowel obstruction, brain metastases) require specific treatment
Sleep	Lack of sleep may be due to other symptoms e.g. pain or anxiety, or be longstanding. Sedatives may help
Low mood/anxiety	Eliciting and addressing concerns, talking therapy, antidepressants or anxiolytics
Appetite and mouth	Can sometimes be helped by adjustment of medication and mouth care, and simple dietary advice. Ill-fitting dentures are a common consequence of weight loss in older people
Breathlessness	Treatment of the underlying cause if possible. Relaxation techniques, a fan, oxygen if hypoxaemic, and careful titration of morphine or benzodiazepines are other measures
Fatigue	Can be a serious problem. Lifestyle adaptation, antidepressants (if low mood) or dexamethasone may help
Relationships, social support and housing	May need help and adaptations at home – involve social services and occupational therapist
Spiritual needs	Offer information about available support if wanted
Any other concerns/things the person wants to do but cannot	For example, this may be something as simple as wanting to go out and visit somewhere, and a wheelchair might allow this

Ask patients to prioritise their problems. Sometimes what is important to the doctor is not the most important thing to the patient.

living allowance if their life expectancy is thought to be less than 6 months. Eligibility for some continuing care packages is dependent on a life expectancy of weeks.

The ability of health professionals to predict survival is known to be poor. In cancer patients, doctors are usually over-optimistic, but predictions become more accurate as death

Box 12.4 **Tips – symptom management in palliative care includes:**

- Thorough assessment, including the patient's perspective. Consider whether the problem is:
  - related to the underlying disease(s)
  - related to the treatment for the disease(s)
  - a co-incidental problem (e.g. angina, arthritis)
  - all of the above? Expect to find multiple causes
- Establishing a realistic management plan with the patient and the rest of the team, and revising the plan as necessary
  - Is the underlying cause treatable?
  - What is the likelihood of success of any treatment?
  - Is the treatment appropriate on the basis of the balance of risks versus benefits for this individual?
  - What is the likely timescale in which improvement will take place?
  - What degree of improvement can be expected?
  - What other options will be available?
- Considering different routes of administration of drugs
  - Although the oral route is preferable, there are several other routes of administration that are used in palliative care, including subcutaneous, rectal, transdermal and transmucosal
- Regular re-assessment, timed according to the severity of the symptom. If symptoms persist, reconsider diagnosis, and route of drug administration. Also remember:
  - treatment of a severe symptom may unmask other symptoms
  - new and evolving symptoms are to be expected in progressive disease
  - ineffective medication should be stopped
- Anticipation of problems – for example, malignant hypercalcaemia usually recurs
- Remembering that mechanical problems require mechanical solutions
  - Constipation secondary to complete tumour obstruction of the rectum will not respond to laxatives and a colostomy may be required

Adapted from Kite S, O'Doherty C. (2007) *Palliative Care*. In: Rai, Mulley, eds. Elderly Medicine: a Training Guide. Elsevier, London.

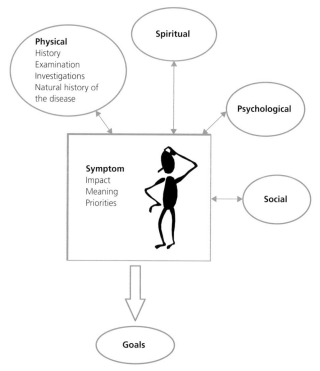

Figure 12.4 Symptoms can be the result of several factors. The aetiology of symptoms ranges from simple to complex. Complex symptoms are the result of several factors, and management involves considering the whole picture.

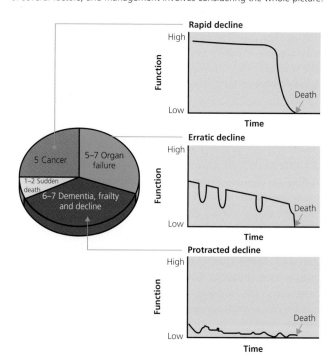

Figure 12.5 Deaths per general practitioner per year and their illness trajectories. Adapted from Keri Thomas (with reference to Joanne Lynn) in Fallon M, Hanks G, eds (2006) *ABC of Palliative Care*, 2nd edn. Blackwell Publishing, Oxford.

approaches. Determining prognosis in non-malignant diseases such as end-stage heart failure and severe chronic obstructive pulmonary disease is even more difficult. These diseases usually have 'entry–re-entry' death trajectories involving acute exacerbations followed by some improvement. Illness trajectories can be useful when looking at prognosis and when trying to match palliative care needs to different patient groups (see Figure 12.5). Box 12.5 lists some prognostic factors in advanced cancer.

Patients often ask, 'How long have I got?' It is helpful to explore why the patient is asking the question now, as a precise answer may be impossible (and sometimes inappropriate), but this provides a useful opportunity to discuss patient expectations, and progress in general, and facilitates the setting of realistic goals.

Box 12.6 summarises a checklist of dos and don'ts in palliative care.

Withdrawing and withholding treatment

The benefits and burdens of treatment need to be reviewed when death is imminent and inevitable. Little is known of the

Box 12.5 **Prognostic factors in advanced cancer**

The following may be useful in estimating prognosis in advanced cancer.
- Clinical judgement
- Performance status of the patient
- The presence of anorexia, weakness and weight loss
- Breathlessness
- Delirium
- Cognitive failure
- Laboratory tests

Some of these factors have been incorporated into validated prognostic scoring systems.

From Maltoni *et al.* (2005) Prognostic factors in advanced cancer patients: evidence-based clinical recommendations. A study by the Steering Committee of the European Association for Palliative Care. *Journal of Clinical Oncology* 23: 6240–8.

Box 12.6 **Dos and don'ts – a checklist for palliative care**

DO
- Elicit patient priorities
- Engage the patient and carers in the management plan
- Set realistic goals
- Try to pre-empt predictable problems whenever possible
- Review progress regularly in view of response, and changing goals
- Stop ineffective medications and interventions
- Plan ahead
- Ensure prompt communication (including the patient) across service boundaries
- Recognise your own limitations and refer on if necessary

DON'T
- Make assumptions about what the patient will want
- Promise things that are not in your control

physiology of dying, but body homeostasis (e.g. whether or not a patient experiences thirst) does appear to be different in the very terminal stages of advanced disease.

If there is uncertainty regarding the potential benefits of a treatment, a therapeutic trial can be undertaken with defined goals and a review date. Making decisions at the end of life requires excellent communication skills, reasonable estimation of prognosis, and teamwork – often the hardest aspects of care. Knowledge of patient wishes and goals in advance helps decision-making, and formal advance decisions can be useful. In the case of patients who have not made advance decisions and who are unable to communicate their wishes or who lack capacity, the views of carers and relatives regarding the patient's likely wishes must be sought. Decisions must be made within the framework of the law and professional guidance (see further resources section).

Cardiopulmonary resuscitation

Decisions regarding cardiopulmonary resuscitation (CPR) can be particularly challenging. Sensitivity is required, and an informed decision made by a competent patient requires realistic information about their prognosis, likelihood of success, and the risks of the procedure.

Older hospital inpatients at best have a 10% chance of surviving to discharge after CPR. For oncology patients there is a survival rate of less than 1% in those who are bed bound with multiple organ failure unresponsive to medical treatment.

Doctors are not obliged to provide treatments that will not work. However, exploration of the patient's expectations and wishes regarding potentially life-sustaining treatments is part of establishing direction, location and goals of care. Studies in older people have shown that preference for CPR is strongly influenced by the perceived probability of surviving a CPR attempt. The majority of patients think that resuscitation is successful most of the time. However, when presented with accurate survival statistics, the number of people who choose CPR falls.

Bereavement

Bereavement has serious health consequences for many people, with up to one-third developing depression. Older people may be even more susceptible for a number of reasons.
- Negative life events are the most important risk factor for depression in older people.
- Poor health, reduced mobility and sensory loss make it more difficult to rebuild an identity or take on new roles.
- Social isolation.
- Lack of employment to buffer the strain of a stressful life event.
- Dementia can reduce the capacity to understand what has happened.

Bereavement support should be offered proactively to those considered most at risk. This includes those lacking social support, those whose history or personality indicate a risk of prolonged grief or circumstances where the events surrounding the death were especially distressing.

Further resources

Fallon M, Hanks G, eds. (2006) *ABC of Palliative Care*, 2nd edn. Blackwell Publishing, Oxford.

Kite S, O'Doherty C. (2007) Palliative care. In: Rai GS, Mulley GP, eds. *Elderly Medicine: a Training Guide*. Elsevier, London.

Twycross R, Wilcock A. (2007) *Palliative Care Formulary*, 3rd edn. www.palliativedrugs.com

British Medical Association. (2007) *Withholding and Withdrawing Life-Prolonging Medical Treatment. Guidance for Decision Making*, 3rd edn. BMA, London.

Decisions relating to cardiopulmonary resuscitation. A joint statement from the British Medical Association, the Resuscitation Council (UK) and the Royal College of Nursing (Oct 2007). www.bma.org.uk/ap.nsf/Content/CPRDecisions07

CHAPTER 13

Discharge Planning

Mamoun Elmamoun & Graham Mulley

OVERVIEW

- Discharge planning starts on admission to hospital
- It involves gathering information about social circumstances and function
- It requires good communication between the multidisciplinary team, relatives, carers and community services
- Discharge summaries should be sent as soon as possible after the patient has left hospital
- There are many barriers to a successful discharge, but a well co-ordinated multidisciplinary team can overcome these

Box 13.1 **Successful discharge planning**

Successful discharge planning involves the following.
- Assessing the patient: to determine his or her medical, social, psychological and functional needs
- Discussion with the family or care givers: their ability to care for the patient, whether they are under strain, whether care services will be needed, and the carers' educational needs are met
- Sharing information with the patient, family and other team members
- Implementation of the plan: arranging for the provision of services and equipment
- Follow-up: the evaluation stage provides feedback that enables the effectiveness of the discharge process to be measured

Definitions

Discharge planning is the process by which the hospital team, liaising with relatives and carers, community services and general practitioners, organises the return of patients to their homes or transfer to other places of care. It is often a multidisciplinary process, which ensures that patients spend no unnecessary time in hospital. Some discharges can be time-consuming and complex. The keys to a successful discharge are information gathering, sharing this information, and planning (Box 13.1). Every detail needs to be considered, especially if the patient has several different problems.

The discharge planning process

Discharge planning starts on admission, by collecting information from the patient and relatives and/or carers about social circumstances and function. It includes a risk assessment for those who are frail or cognitively impaired, or have inadequate social support. It prepares the patient, relatives, multidisciplinary team and other healthcare providers for a safe and efficient discharge back to the pre-admission destination or suitable alternative. The stages of discharge planning are shown in Figure 13.1.

Discharge planning involves good communication:
- with the patient and relatives or carers, whose active involvement is central to the success of the discharge

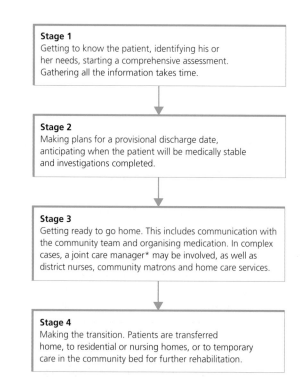

Stage 1
Getting to know the patient, identifying his or her needs, starting a comprehensive assessment. Gathering all the information takes time.

Stage 2
Making plans for a provisional discharge date, anticipating when the patient will be medically stable and investigations completed.

Stage 3
Getting ready to go home. This includes communication with the community team and organising medication. In complex cases, a joint care manager* may be involved, as well as district nurses, community matrons and home care services.

Stage 4
Making the transition. Patients are transferred home, to residential or nursing homes, or to temporary care in the community bed for further rehabilitation.

Figure 13.1 The stages of discharge planning.

*A joint care manager is a person with a nursing or social work background who deals with people who require both health and social care in the community.

ABC of Geriatric Medicine. Edited by N. Cooper, K. Forrest and G. Mulley.
© 2009 Blackwell Publishing, ISBN: 978-1-4051-6942-4.

64

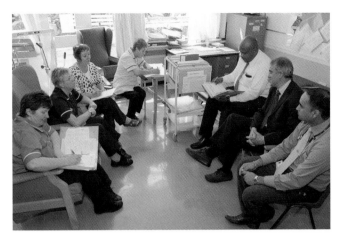

Figure 13.2 A typical weekly multidisciplinary team meeting.

- within the ward-based multidisciplinary team (e.g. at formal meetings, during ward rounds or at other times). See Figure 13.2.
- between the ward staff and members of the community team.

The different members of the multidisciplinary team are shown in Box 13.2.

Comprehensive geriatric assessment

Patients identified as high risk (e.g. recurrent falls, dementia, struggling at home) should have a comprehensive geriatric assessment (see Chapter 1). In the context of discharge planning, this involves the following.

- Medical assessment and treatment.
- Review of medicines and concordance (see Chapter 2).
- Gathering information about social circumstances, including details of carers, social services, benefits and whether there is any carer strain.
- Assessment of cognitive function, including the patient's ability to participate in discharge planning, and if not, identifying a representative.
- Assessment of functional ability (i.e. ability to perform activities of daily living and instrumental – or extended – activities of daily living which is helpful in assessing a patient's need for rehabilitation or support – see Box 13.3).
- Asking about living arrangements (e.g. whether there are stairs at home).
- Formulating goals, which should be specific and agreed with the patient, relatives and carers.
- Eliciting patient preferences about discharge plans.

Following this, referrals may be made to social services or mental health teams. Physiotherapy and occupational therapy input may be needed. An estimation of when patients will be medically fit is made – this may include when they will be ready to go to a rehabilitation facility, if needed.

The single assessment process (SAP)

The SAP brings together health and social services information in a single document. It aims to improve communication between

healthcare and social care workers, in theory allowing services to be more responsive to the patient's needs. It avoids the patient having to repeat the same information to a range of professionals and is started in hospital if the patient does not have one already. The file follows the patient. The language used is clear and concise, avoiding jargon and abbreviations.

Box 13.2 Different members of the multidisciplinary team (MDT)

Team members	Role
Doctors	Assess, diagnose, treat and review medical conditions A consultant geriatrician often 'chairs' the MDT meetings
Nurses	Nursing care, gather information about home circumstances and function, assess patient, work with other MDT members, co-ordinate discharge planning
Physiotherapists	Assess and treat movement disorders, often using physical therapies, in order to restore function, mobility and independence
Occupational therapists	Assess patient's ability to perform activities of daily living, assess risk (e.g. in the kitchen) and recommend interventions to help maximise participation and independence
Dieticians	Assess and recommend treatment for nutritional status
Speech and language therapists	Assess and recommend treatment for disorders of speech, language and swallowing
Pharmacists	Check medication list, assess concordance, educate patients, give advice about new medicines
Social workers/joint care managers	Assess need for care (using reports from the rest of the MDT) versus current health and social care package. May also review finances and assist with a change of living arrangements. Also advises on benefits or legal issues
Specialist nurses, podiatry, intermediate care teams, mental health teams, community matrons, general practitioners, palliative care teams	According to patient need

The MDT is a group of professionals who work together and take responsibility for patient care and discharge planning. The core of the MDT consists of doctors, nurses, physiotherapist, occupational therapist, pharmacist and a social worker or joint care manager.

Box 13.3 **Activities of daily living (ADL) and instrumental activities of daily living (IADL)**

Activities of daily living (ADLs)	Instrumental activities of daily living (IADLs)
Bathing	Preparing meals
Dressing	Shopping
Eating	Using the telephone
Toileting	Doing housework
Mobility and transfers	Taking medication
	Managing money

Good practice with medications

A review of medicines and concordance is usually done by a pharmacist. Medicine aids can be helpful in improving compliance. Examples are:

- Dosette box – a plastic refillable box with labels for the days of the week and time of day, filled by the patient or their relatives/carers
- blister pack – like a Dossette box only heat-sealed and prepared under the direct supervision of a pharmacist.

Prescriptions should be explained to the patient and/or carers, highlighting any changes since admission (see Figure 13.3). They should also be informed about important side-effects. Inadequate preparation is associated with adverse events. Patients who are unable to remember a discussion about the side-effects of their medication are at a threefold greater risk of experiencing an adverse event than patients who can recall such information.

Home visits and equipment

Visiting the home with or without the patient, either before or on the day of discharge, can provide hospital or community staff with the opportunity to identify problems, as well as addressing any other needs that the patient and/or carers may have. Home visits are done in selected complex patients by occupational therapists and physiotherapists (see Figure 13.4).

Occupational therapists also determine if the patient would benefit from equipment or modifications in the home. They decide whether any previously provided equipment is still suitable and if any new aids, appliances or environmental adjustments (e.g. Telecare – see Chapter 14) are required.

Discharge summaries

The discharge summary is an important communication tool. It provides key information about admission, diagnosis, investigations, interventions and follow-up arrangements. It is useful for healthcare providers to implement the treatment strategies planned during admission, thus ensuring effective continuity of care in the community. However, many summaries omit information on cognition (e.g. Mini Mental State Examination score) and function (ability to perform activities of daily living).

It is important that discharge summaries are clear, complete and sent to the general practitioner and care home at the earliest opportunity (ideally within a few days, although organisational

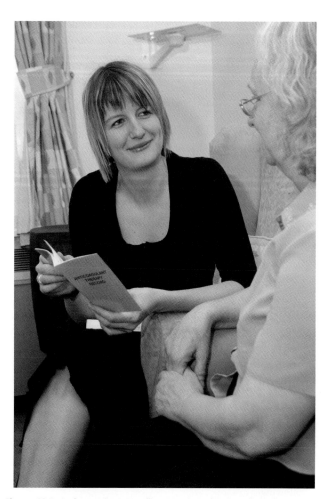

Figure 13.3 A pharmacist counselling a patient about warfarin therapy.

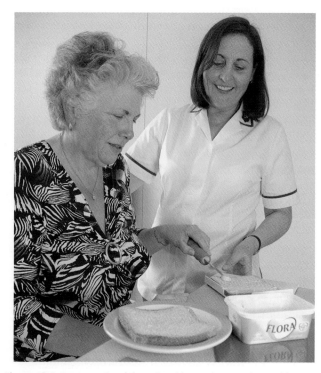

Figure 13.4 An occupational therapist with a patient on a home visit.

Box 13.4 **Checklist for a discharge summary**

- Hospital, ward, consultant and contact numbers
- Patient's name and unique identifier (i.e. hospital number, date of birth and address)
- Date of admission and date of discharge
- Discharge destination (which may not be home)
- Problem list
- Clinical story including significant investigation results
- What information has been given to the patient and family
- Functional and cognitive status on discharge
- What follow-up is required or has been arranged
- Medication list, with an explanation of changes

If the patient has been discharged to a care home, or an intermediate care bed, a copy of the discharge summary should also be sent to the attending doctor there.

Box 13.5 **Types of suboptimal discharge**

- Too soon
- Delayed
- To unsafe environments
- To inappropriate environments (e.g. premature discharge to long-term care)
- Poorly organised (e.g. not meeting the patient's and relatives/carers' needs or expectations)

problems often mean this does not occur). A comprehensive discharge summary should contain the information shown in Box 13.4.

Problems in discharge planning

Fragmentation of care can occur if different specialties are involved or if the patient has been moved from ward to ward. Further difficulties can arise when:

- patients and relatives/carers are not fully involved in discharge plans
- patients and relatives/carers do not co-operate with assessments (e.g. physiotherapy or giving information to the social worker)
- there is conflict about the preferred destination on discharge
- there is patchy availability of community services
- patients, relatives/carers or staff want discharge to occur before the patient is medically fit
- ward teams are understaffed or poorly trained and not enough time is given to planning discharge properly (see Box 13.5).

Delayed discharges

A delayed discharge occurs when a multidisciplinary team decision has been made that the patient is ready for discharge from a hospital bed but the patient is still occupying that bed. An unfortunate term for this is 'bed-blocking' – a term that blames

the patient for what is an organisational problem. Delayed discharges have a direct and negative impact on the quality of care for patients. For example, if they stay in an acute ward once their medical needs have been met, they may lose their independence, mobility and social networks, and are at risk of falls and hospital-acquired infections. For patients with dementia, there are additional risks of losing capacity and of premature entry into a care home.

Recurrent admissions

Patients who frequently attend hospitals are a vulnerable heterogeneous group – a mixture of patients with chronic medical, mental health and psychosocial problems. The inelegant term 'frequent flyer' is used to describe such individuals. Most re-admissions are the result of a new medical problem, exacerbation of an existing problem, or care-giver difficulties. Multidisciplinary teams and community matrons have been introduced in many areas to see if improved community care for such people can prevent admissions to hospital. Hospital-acquired infections may become evident only after patients have gone home, so information about what to look out for and whom to call is useful. Follow-up plans should also be clear, otherwise patients can inadvertently 'slip through the net'.

Carer strain

Carers often provide a vital role in supporting patients at home. Many carers find their role fulfilling, but caring can be an exhausting task. 'Red flags' that can identify situations in which there is potential carer strain include sleep disturbance, faecal incontinence and behavioural problems on the part of the patient.

Conclusions

The key to a successful discharge is good communication between individuals and teams. This includes patients, their relatives/carers, hospital and community services. Box 13.6 provides some further tips.

Box 13.6 **Tips for a successful discharge**

- Make no assumptions (e.g. that families can provide care, that family members agree with each other)
- Keep up to date with developments from other members of the multidisciplinary team – often new information comes to light which changes the original discharge plan
- Review the patient on the day of discharge, to ensure there is no new medical problem
- Ensure that patients are discharged only when necessary equipment and services are in place
- Ensure that the preliminary discharge summary (usually written by a junior doctor) is clear, comprehensive and correct
- Telephone the general practitioner before discharge if the patient is terminally ill or requires medical monitoring in the early days after discharge

Further resources

Department of Health. (2003) *Discharge from Hospital: Pathway, Process and Practice.* DH, London. www.dh.gov.uk

Scottish Intercollegiate Guidelines Network. (2002) *Management of Patients with Stroke: Rehabilitation, Prevention and Management of Complications, and Discharge Planning.* A national clinical guideline [no 64]. SIGN, Edinburgh. www.sign.ac.uk

Bull MJ, Roberts J. Components of a proper hospital discharge for elders. *J Adv Nur*s 2001; 35: 571–81.

Cooper N, Forrest K, Cramp P. (2006) Medical records. In: *Essential Guide to Generic Skills.* Blackwell Publishing, Oxford.

Acknowledgements

The authors wish to thank the many people in the Leeds Teaching Hospitals and Primary Care Trusts who have contributed to this chapter.

CHAPTER 14

Intermediate Care

Nicola Turner & Catherine Tandy

OVERVIEW

- Intermediate care aims to promote faster recovery from illness, maximise independence, and prevent unnecessary time in hospital
- The single assessment process is documentation that facilitates assessment of people's needs without duplication by different agencies
- Community matrons proactively manage patients with long-term conditions
- There are increasing initiatives to improve advanced planning of care, particularly end of life care, in the community

---

Box 14.1 **Definition of intermediate care**

The Department of Health definition, supported by the British Geriatrics Society, states that the term 'intermediate care' describes services that meet all of the following criteria.
- Targeted at people who would otherwise have had an unnecessarily prolonged hospital stay, or inappropriate admission to acute inpatient care, long-term residential care, or continuing NHS inpatient care
- Provided on the basis of a comprehensive assessment, resulting in a structured individual care plan that involves active therapy, treatment and opportunity for recovery
- Has a planned outcome of maximising independence and typically enabling patients to resume living at home
- Is time limited, typically no longer than 6 weeks and frequently as little as 1 or 2 weeks
- Involves cross-professional working, with a single assessment framework, single professional records and shared protocols

Intermediate care – the context

The development of intermediate care services first became UK Department of Health policy with the publication of the National Health Service (NHS) Plan in 2000. The National Service Framework for Older People followed in 2001, setting out targets and goals for the introduction of intermediate care services. In 2004, the NHS Improvement Plan introduced the new role of community matrons to support patients with long-term conditions at home.

In 2006, *Our Health, Our Care, Our Say: a New Direction for Community Services* was published and set out the government's vision for integration of health and social care services, and providing more care closer to people's homes. The clinical case supporting these changes was set out by the National Director for Older People in his 2007 report *A Recipe for Care – Not a Single Ingredient.*

In response to these agendas, intermediate care services have been developed. Community matrons have been appointed. Increasing numbers of consultant geriatricians now work in the community as well as the acute hospital. Teams are working to support older people in the community, including palliative and end of life care.

What is intermediate care?

Intermediate care is a range of integrated services provided at or near to a person's home that aims to promote faster recovery from illness, maximise independence, prevent unnecessary admission to hospital and facilitate timely discharge (see Box 14.1). It allows appropriate and early access to comprehensive geriatric assessment and involves working across health and social care boundaries.

Services at the interface between hospital and primary care have developed in response to national policies and local needs. This has resulted in geographical variations in local implementation and different models of intermediate care (Box 14.2). Many areas run a combination of models. Composition of teams and leadership of services also varies (Box 14.3). Services may be led by nurses, general practitioners or geriatricians.

Why is intermediate care important?

Intermediate care offers a co-ordinated service that links primary and acute hospital care, community health services, social care, carer support and health promotion. It makes more effective use of hospital capacity and consequently helps support waiting time targets and allows better response to emergency and seasonal pressures.

Evaluation of intermediate care services has demonstrated reduced length of stay in hospital and higher patient satisfaction ratings. Outcomes are at least as good as traditional acute hospital care and costs are roughly equivalent. Intermediate care may also

ABC of Geriatric Medicine. Edited by N. Cooper, K. Forrest and G. Mulley. © 2009 Blackwell Publishing, ISBN: 978-1-4051-6942-4.

Box 14.2 **Different models of intermediate care**

Residential rehabilitation	Intermediate care based in care in community beds. These beds may be located in a care home or community hospital close to the patient's home
Home-based rehabilitation	Intermediate care based in the patient's home
Hospital at home	Provide active treatment by healthcare professionals in the patient's own home for a condition that would otherwise require acute inpatient care. Examples include the administration of intravenous antibiotics
Early discharge schemes	These target groups of patients with a specific condition for an early supported discharge from hospital e.g. patients with stroke or chronic obstructive pulmonary disease
Day hospital	Provides a variety of multidisciplinary therapy, medical investigations and treatment. Access to specialist clinics may also be available e.g. falls or continence clinics
Rapid response teams	Respond to referrals from ambulance services, the emergency department, general practitioners, community nurses and social services. They allow rapid assessment and identification of patients' needs and facilitate appropriate care and rehabilitation in the community

Box 14.3 **The intermediate care team**

- Nurses
- Physiotherapists
- Occupational therapists
- Care support workers
- Social worker/joint care manager
- Doctor – geriatrician or general practitioner with a special interest (GPwSI)
- Others, e.g. pharmacist, community psychiatric nurse

reduce the need for long-term residential care by allowing time and space for recovery of health and independence before decisions are made about future care needs.

The single assessment process

The single assessment process (SAP), described in Chapter 13, is central to intermediate care provision. It is documentation that facilitates a thorough assessment of people's needs without duplication by different agencies. Examples of documentation tools include:
- EASY-Care
- Camberwell Assessment for the Needs of the Elderly (CANE)
- Functional Assessment of the Care Environment (FACE).

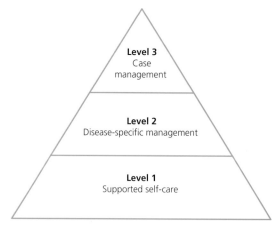

Level 1 Appropriate for the majority of people with long-term conditions. Work with patients and carers to develop knowledge, skills and confidence to care for themselves and their condition

Level 2 High-risk patients with complex single needs cared for by multidisciplinary teams and disease-specific protocols and pathways (e.g. severe chronic obstructive pulmonary disease or heart failure)

Level 3 Requires identification of highly complex patients who are very high users of emergency care. Community matron or other professional to use case management approach to anticipate, co-ordinate and join up health and social care

Figure 14.1 Models of care in the community.

Use of SAP is not unique to intermediate care. The vision is for hospital and community health providers to use the same documentation along with social care agencies, enabling sharing of information to best meet the needs of the individual.

Community matrons and long-term conditions

Patients with long-term conditions (chronic diseases) are high users of NHS resources, requiring a large number of visits to their general practitioner and often frequent admissions to hospital. Community matrons have been introduced to take a proactive approach to chronic disease management for the most complex patients, instead of the previous reactive pattern of healthcare. Their roles have been developed from models of care in the United States by companies such as Kaiser Permanente and Evercare (see Figure 14.1).

Patients needing the support of a matron are identified using various tools designed to predict future likelihood of hospital admission. These are based on the number of conditions and previous admission rates. The most commonly used is the PARR tool (Patients At Risk of Readmission) developed by the King's Fund and partners (see Box 14.4). The decision algorithms are constantly being refined following ongoing research, to improve their case-finding accuracy. The main drawback of the currently available versions is that they use an acute admission as the trigger for analysis and identification and give weight to the number of previous admissions. At present there are no tools to help identify those who have not yet had several admissions but will go on to do so in the future.

Community matrons are experienced nurses trained in chronic disease management, including skills in history taking, clinical

Box 14.4 **Data included in the PARR tool**

Demographics	Age
	Gender
	Ethnicity
	Postcode
Hospital use	Diagnostic codes
	Specialities involved
	Number of admissions
	Emergency department
	attendances
Community characteristics	Local age- and sex-adjusted rates
	of hospitalisation for conditions
Hospital of current admission	Admission practices of local
	hospital specialists

examination and prescribing. They provide a holistic assessment of the patient's needs. By visiting the person regularly in their own home, they are able to build up a full picture of the individual, incorporating physical, psychological, social and family dimensions, all of which have an impact on healthcare use. They act as co-ordinators of the various agencies involved in the individual's care and facilitate access to specialist teams and social support networks where appropriate.

Community matrons work alongside general practitioners and hospital specialists to ensure that management of chronic disease is optimised. They teach patients and carers how to self-manage their condition whenever possible. Regular monitoring allows early detection of exacerbations, frequently at a stage when treatment can be successfully modified in the community, in theory avoiding an acute admission to hospital.

Psychological problems are a common trigger for acute admission when there is no objective change in the patient's physical status. A common example is anxiety in breathless patients with chronic lung disease. Community matrons build a trusting relationship with their patients and can help alleviate these problems by giving people time to talk through their concerns, as well as accessing anxiety management therapy where appropriate.

Telecare

Used in combination with other services, telecare systems use a variety of assistive technologies and monitoring devices to maintain safety and allow access in order to support patients' independence in the home. Sophisticated adaptations are possible that allow people with extremely limited physical function to operate domestic appliances independently using computer controls. However, these systems are complex and expensive and are usually reserved for younger disabled people. For older people, telecare equipment assists in the care of patients with cognitive impairment using such things as door entry systems, pendant alarms, automated medication prompt devices, fall detectors and movement sensors.

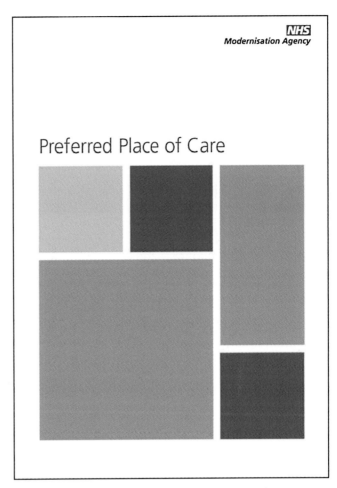

Figure 14.2 Preferred place of care document. Contains guidance to facilitate patients' choice regarding end of life care in their own home, hospice or care home.

Advanced care planning and end of life care

There are increasing initiatives to improve advanced planning of care, particularly end of life care, in the community. Community matrons and other staff are being encouraged to use 'preferred place of care' documentation with their service users. This facilitates discussion of the patients' wishes regarding their care in the future, specifically where they wish to be cared for at the end of life. Research suggests that most patients want to die at home, but currently the majority die in hospital.

The preferred place of care document (Figure 14.2) is a form of advance directive, also known as a 'living will', which allows people to state their wishes while they are able to do so, in order that those caring for them know what they would have wanted when they are no longer able to participate in decision-making. Advance directives take many forms, from specific instructions about advance refusal of a particular treatment, to values statements about what is important to the individual's quality of life.

The NHS End of Life Care Programme (Figure 14.3), the Gold Standards Framework (GSF) mentioned in Chapter 12 (Figure 14.4), and similar initiatives are gradually being introduced to further individual and their family when death is near. These initiatives were first introduced for patients at home but are now being extended to people in care homes.

Tools such as the Liverpool Care Pathway for the Dying, commonly used in hospital environments, are increasingly being used in a form adapted for community use. This improves end of life care by prompting staff to systematically address all aspects of care. This includes withdrawal of unnecessary medications and ensuring drugs are prescribed for symptom control, including for symptoms that are likely to develop. In addition there are prompts to ensure spiritual needs have been met as well as bereavement care for the family.

Long-term care

One aim of geriatric medicine, and community services in particular, is to maintain older people in their own homes for as long as possible. However, inevitably some do need long-term care in residential or nursing homes. Currently there is little systematic care for these individuals and standards vary widely. In some areas, general practitioners undertake regular visits to care homes. In other areas, community matrons are starting to provide support and advice to residents and care home staff. Community geriatricians are also beginning to increase their involvement in care homes.

Further resources

British Geriatrics Society. *Intermediate Care: Guidance for Commissioners and Providers of Health and Social Care.* BGS Compendium Document 4.2, revised 2004. www.bgs.org.uk

Department of Health. (2007) *A Recipe for Care – Not a Single Ingredient.* Clinical case for change: report by Professor Ian Philp, National Director for Older People. DH, London. www.dh.gov.uk

British Geriatrics Society. (2005) *Geriatricians and the Management of Long-Term Conditions. Report of the Primary and Continuing Care Special Interest Group.* BGS, London. www.bgs.org.uk

Mulley GP. (2006) Intermediate or indeterminate care: evidence-based community rehabilitation. The Marjorie Robertson Lecture at the 44th St Andrew's Festival Symposium on geriatric medicine. *J R Coll Physicians Edin* 36. www.rcpe.ac.uk/publications/articles/July_06/240505_A_MUL.pdf

Young J, Sykes A. The evidence base for intermediate care. *CME Geriat Med* 2005; 7(3): 117–25.

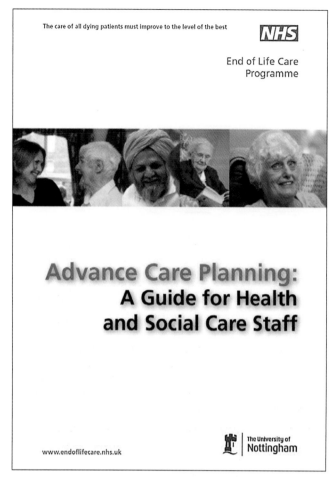

Figure 14.3 The document *Advanced Care Planning: A Guide for Health and Social Care Staff.* Contains guidance on advanced planning regarding end of life care with patients who have life-limiting conditions. www.endoflifecare.nhs.uk

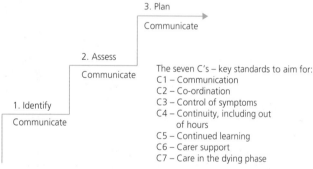

Figure 14.4 The Gold Standards Framework.

improve palliative care. The GSF provides a plan to assist primary care organisations to develop a palliative care register where patients nearing the end of life are identified before the final terminal stage. This allows time for their needs and wishes to be defined and planned so that systems are in place to properly support the

CHAPTER 15

Benefits and Social Services

John Pearn & Rosemary Young

OVERVIEW

- Old people are more likely to have low incomes
- Many pensioners do not claim all the benefits to which they are entitled
- Family members provide the majority of social care provided in the community
- There is a range of statutory services and benefits available to older people
- The Mental Capacity Act (2005) allows people to make a lasting power of attorney, so that a designated person (the attorney) can make decisions about their property, affairs and personal welfare

Box 15.1 **Older people and income**

- State benefits are the main source of income for pensioners
- Older pensioners generally have less wealth than those around retirement age
- At least half a million pensioners do not claim the benefits to which they are entitled
- Spending priorities change with age, with an increasing proportion of total spending going on food, housing and fuel
- In 2001 a third of older households lived in poor housing and this proportion increased with age. The most common reason for a dwelling to be declared inadequate was insufficient heating

Information from the Office for National Statistics. www.statistics.gov.uk

Old people in society

Old people are more likely to have low incomes and problems with housing (see Box 15.1). Although there is a wide range of statutory services and benefits available, many older people have a limited understanding of their entitlements. Indeed, many health professionals are unfamiliar with the full range of services available. This may serve as a barrier to older people claiming benefits or services for which they are eligible.

Only about 5% of older people live in institutions, although this figure rises to 25% in those aged over 85 (see Figure 15.1). Most elderly people live independently at home, with over half of women over the age of 75 living alone. There are estimated to be 6 million informal carers in the UK, many of whom are pensioners themselves (see Figure 15.2). The physical, emotional, financial and social strain placed upon some carers is therefore a significant problem.

Benefits

All people over the age of 65 who have paid sufficient national insurance contributions are eligible for a state pension in the UK. If their weekly income falls below a minimum threshold a top-up pension credit may be payable. Those on a low income may be able to claim housing benefit to cover part or all of their rent, and council

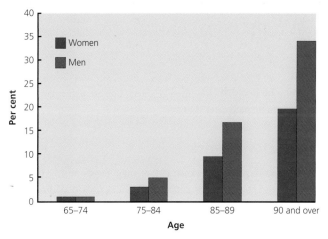

Figure 15.1 People who live in care homes, by age and sex (April 2001, Great Britain). Information from the Office for National Statistics. www.statistics.gov.uk

tax credit to the value of all or part of their council tax liability. Winter fuel payments are made to those aged over 60 to cover the additional costs of heating during winter months.

Attendance allowance may be paid to people aged over 65 to help meet the cost of paying for personal care (e.g. help with washing, dressing and getting in or out of bed). Disability living allowance is a similar benefit payable to younger adults living with a chronic disability. Mobility allowance can be claimed for the

ABC of Geriatric Medicine. Edited by N. Cooper, K. Forrest and G. Mulley.
© 2009 Blackwell Publishing, ISBN: 978-1-4051-6942-4.

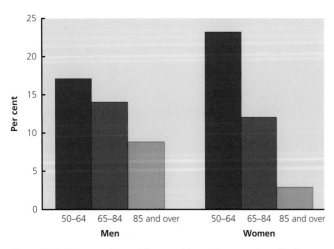

Figure 15.2 Older people providing unpaid care, by sex and age (April 2001, England and Wales). Information from the Office for National Statistics. www.statistics.gov.uk

---

Box 15.2 How clinicians can help carers

- Recognise and acknowledge the role of the informal carer
- Listen to carers – they know the person they care for very well. When taking a social history, specifically enquire about how they are coping
- Give information about diagnosis and prognosis
- Make available information about statutory, voluntary and private provision of services in your area, including respite care
- Direct carers towards sources of information and support (see further resources section)

---

first time by people below the age of 65, but once granted it may continue to be paid after that age.

Supporting carers

Carers may request an assessment of their needs at any time. In England and Wales carers can have services provided directly to them, which may be subject to means testing. In Scotland, carers cannot receive services in their own right, but their needs should be taken into account when assessing the person they care for. Home adaptations and help with caring and household tasks may be available. Sitting services can allow carers to leave the house for a few hours at a time, or respite care may allow them to take a longer break. There is a number of voluntary organisations providing support and advice for carers (see further resources section) and there are a number of ways in which clinicians can help (Box 15.2).

Carers' allowance is a means-tested benefit payable to those caring for a chronically disabled person for at least 35 hours a week. To be eligible, the carer's income must be below a minimum threshold, and the disabled person must be receiving either an attendance allowance or disability living allowance.

Box 15.3 A typical case history

An 83-year-old lady was admitted following a fall at home. A diagnosis of a urinary tract infection with a background of dementia was made. She lived alone in her own property, and had been widowed 2 years ago. She received regular support from her daughter, but did not have a formal package of care. Her mobility had declined in recent years, and she sometimes had difficulty reaching the toilet in time. Her daughter assisted with shopping, but often found out-of-date food in the fridge. She seemed disinclined to prepare her own meals, and ate mainly soup or sandwiches.

Before discharge, a comprehensive geriatric assessment was performed, including assessments by physiotherapists, occupational therapists, nursing staff and social workers. A care plan was made.

- The council installed grab rails at her front door, on the stairs and in the bathroom, and a downstairs commode was provided
- A local voluntary organisation could deliver meals on wheels, and Age Concern provided contact details for a local luncheon club
- Home care was arranged, to assist with bathing and medication prompts in the mornings. Costs were met in part by the local authority, and partly by the patient herself
- The social worker advised that she could claim attendance allowance to cover the cost of employing a carer
- Since her basic state pension fell below the minimum threshold, she was also eligible to receive pension credit and council tax credit

---

Statutory services

Any older person has the right to request a social services care assessment. This may be focused upon meeting specific needs, such as home adaptations, or a more general multidisciplinary team assessment may be required. Following the assessment, a care plan is agreed, and a care manager appointed to act as a liaison between the patient and social services. Care may be provided by a number of different agencies. Social services provide care that meets primarily social rather than healthcare needs – for example, assistance with toileting, bathing or dressing. Voluntary organisations may provide meals on wheels, day centres or luncheon clubs. Care designed to meet medical needs, such as the administration of medication or the care of pressure areas, is funded by the National Health Service (NHS). Some people may choose to accept direct cash payments, to enable them to purchase their own choice of care services. Box 15.3 illustrates a typical case history.

There are regional variations in the extent to which service users are expected to fund their own care. In Scotland personal care is free to those aged over 65; in Northern Ireland home help services are provided free to the over 75s; in England and Wales, a means-tested contribution may be payable and each local council sets its own charging policy, in accordance with national guidelines.

Continuing care

Continuing healthcare is funded primarily by the NHS rather than by social services, and is appropriate for people who have ongoing medical needs requiring care delivered by, or under the supervision of, registered healthcare practitioners. Care may be delivered in

Box 15.4 **Levels of continuing care**

- **Level 1** – suitable for those requiring assistance with activities of daily living, or intervention from a trained nurse on an intermittent and predictable basis.
- **Level 2** – suitable for those requiring 24-hour supervision, but not necessarily the constant presence of a registered nurse.
- **Level 3** – suitable for those requiring primarily accommodation and social care, but who have co-existing medical needs requiring the constant availability of trained nursing staff.
- **Level 4** – suitable for those requiring either a short-term specialist rehabilitation assessment, or long-term rehabilitation.
- **Level 5** – suitable for those with complex or unpredictable physical or mental health needs who require frequent intervention, treatment or supervision by a healthcare professional. Examples include patients with challenging behaviour or frequent seizures, or those in a persistent vegetative state.
- **Level 6** – suitable for patients in the final stages of life, with a prognosis not expected to exceed a matter of weeks. They may require specialised palliative care, and high-intensity nursing. Provided there is agreement that care can be delivered safely, patients may choose to receive care in any setting, including their own home.

Box 15.5 **Levels of care home**

Residential home care is suitable for those who require mainly social care, with minimal or stable medical needs that do not require the continual presence of registered nursing staff. The residents:
- must be mobile with equipment
- only need the help or supervision of one person for activities of daily living
- may be incontinent of urine or have a urinary catheter
- may have cognitive impairment without challenging behaviour.

Nursing home care is suitable for those with more complex medical needs requiring the 24-hour presence of registered nursing staff. The residents:
- may be immobile
- are dependent for all care
- have unstable medical conditions, such as severe chronic obstructive pulmonary disease requiring oxygen therapy, problematic diabetes or palliative care conditions
- may be fed by percutaneous gastrostomy tube.

Elderly mentally infirm (EMI) care is required if a person's behaviour is challenging, or for those prone to dangerous wandering or physical aggression. EMI homes can be either residential or nursing, although EMI beds are in short supply in the UK.

the person's own home, or in a residential or nursing home. There are six levels of funding, banded according to the complexity and intensity of the care required (see Box 15.4).

Moving into a care home

Older adults in England and Wales with the means to pay can choose to move into a care home at any time, applying directly to a home of their choice. Those requiring financial assistance must apply to social services for funding. The first step is to conduct a multidisciplinary assessment of the person's care needs. His or her views, and those of their relatives or carers, are also taken into account.

Funding for a care home placement may be met in full or in part by the local council or from the person's savings. In cases where nursing care is required, the NHS may make a contribution. A financial assessment is performed by a social worker, to assess what contribution, if any, the elderly person should make towards the cost of care. An inventory of assets is taken. Those with savings above a set threshold are expected to meet the full fees. This upper limit varies between regions, but is around £20 000.

If a person owns his own home, its value will be disregarded for the first 12 weeks of a permanent placement. Thereafter, it may be counted as 'capital', and the person may be expected to sell it to pay their fees. An exception may be made if a relative or partner would be made homeless if the property were sold. If the person has chosen to give away property or savings to a relative, these may still be counted as capital unless they were transferred more than 7 years ago.

Once funding arrangements have been agreed, the person and their relatives are invited to choose a home. The home must be willing to enter into a contract with the local council, and be suitable for the person's needs. If the preferred choice of home costs more than the local council would normally expect to pay, the person or the relatives may be asked to make up the difference. Box 15.5 outlines the different levels of care home available.

Mental capacity

Capacity is a legal term, and refers to a person's ability to make decisions or take actions that have legal consequences. Every adult is assumed to have capacity unless there is evidence to the contrary. To have capacity an individual must be able to:
- understand and retain information relevant to the decision
- believe that information
- weigh the information and arrive at a choice
- communicate the decision.

The rejection of medical advice does not mean a lack of capacity. Any adult may choose to refuse any proposed intervention in full or in part, no matter how irrational, illogical or ill-considered their decision may appear.

Capacity may change with time, for example due to delirium or the natural progression of a dementia. The presence of a dementia or mental illness *per se* does not mean a lack of capacity. On a good day a person may be lucid enough to discuss his or her care. In addition, the degree of capacity required depends upon the legal consequences of the decision being made. A person with advanced dementia may have the capacity to refuse to have a wash that day, but not to make a will or sell his or her house.

Any doctor with the appropriate skills can assess a person's capacity. A psychiatric assessment is not necessary except in difficult cases. Social workers, lawyers and healthcare professionals can also

Box 15.6 **The Mental Capacity Act (2005)**

This allows a person with lasting power of attorney to make decisions about personal welfare, as well as property and affairs. Personal welfare includes:

- deciding where the patient will live
- giving or refusing consent to medical treatment on the patient's behalf.

The act is underpinned by five key principles.

- Everyone is presumed to have capacity unless proved otherwise.
- People have the right to be supported and helped to make their own decisions wherever possible.
- People have the right to make what might seem to be unwise or eccentric decisions.
- Decisions made on behalf of another should be made in the person's best interests. The patient's medical, emotional, social, spiritual and financial needs should be taken into account, as should any previously expressed wishes and their right to liberty, quality of life and dignity.
- Decisions made on behalf of another must be the least restrictive of their basic rights and freedoms.

The Act also stipulates that any relevant advance statements must be considered in the decision-making process. This includes advance refusal of life-saving treatment.

Box 15.7 **Powers of attorney**

- An *ordinary* power of attorney can be arranged via your solicitor if you go abroad for a year. It allows someone else to manage your property and financial affairs in your absence, but becomes invalid if you lose the capacity to do so
- An *enduring* power of attorney remains in force if you lose capacity. It is commonly used by older people to empower their relatives to help them manage their affairs and property should they lose capacity, for example in dementia
- A *lasting* power of attorney may manage your property and affairs, *and* take decisions regarding your personal welfare and medical care if you lack capacity to do so

A power of attorney can only be granted by a person who has the capacity to do so. If a person already lacks capacity, an attorney may be appointed by the Court of Protection.

assess capacity. When people are unable to give or withhold consent, healthcare professionals may proceed with any necessary treatment that is in their best interests. Consideration should be given not only to medical interests, but also emotional, social, financial and spiritual interests as well. A person's previously expressed wishes, including any written advanced directives, must also be taken into account.

Before April 2007 in England and Wales, no-one could give consent on behalf of another adult who lacked mental capacity. The role of a person's relatives was therefore restricted to providing background information on previous beliefs, values, and opinions which might have influenced his or her decisions if they had had capacity. However, the Mental Capacity Act (2005) now makes provision for people to appoint a 'lasting power of attorney'. An attorney is empowered to make decisions on the person's behalf, in circumstances when he or she no longer has capacity. This may encompass medical care, as well as social welfare, housing and financial affairs. See Boxes 15.6 and 15.7. Further information on the Mental Capacity Act can also be found in the further resources section.

Further resources

Age Concern – the UK's largest charity working with and for older people. www.ageconcern.org.uk

Help the Aged – an international charity. www.helptheaged.org.uk

Carers UK (formerly the carers' national association) – a carers' support and information network. www.carersuk.org

Alzheimer's Society – a charity for people with dementia and their families and carers. www.alzheimers.org.uk

Cooper N, Forrest K, Cramp P, eds. (2006) Part II Legal and ethical issues in healthcare. In: *Essential Guide to Generic Skills*. Blackwell Publishing, Oxford.

Bartlett P. (2005) *Blackstone's Guide to the Mental Capacity Act 2005*. Oxford University Press, Oxford.

Index